A Place to Start Without Sugar or Starch

Second Edition

Roanne King

www.CSIDRecipes.com

2016

Second Edition

Dedication

I dedicate this book first to my five amazing children; Elora, Tayler, Dawson, Jared and Parker. You are my life and my purpose in everything I do. May this book also serve as a *starting place* for each of you as you begin your lives away from home in the years to come. May you always appreciate your health and never take it for granted!

Next, I dedicate this book to the many CSID families across the globe. I am honored to be able to touch your lives and give you some amount of encouragement. You have walked this journey with me for several years. Thanks for not giving up on my efforts and for believing in me as another mom, just doing the best I can to care for my family.

Roanne King

Table of Contents

Acknowledgements

First of all, I would like to thank God and his ever guiding Holy Spirit for strength, resolve and giving me the ability to press on even in the most hopeless moments. Not until I reach heaven will I ever understand your favor over my life and the lives of my husband and children. I consider it an honor to work diligently on your behalf to serve and encourage other parents in the hope that I may shine a small speck of the light of Jesus into their lives. I cannot deny and will not hide the fact that what I have accomplished in this book is far beyond my capacity as a human alone. This book is nothing but the result of divine intervention, miracles and healing.

To place others in an order of greatest to least in regards to my gratitude is impossible. So please do not consider your placement in this list in any way an indication of how important your role has played in supporting me in this project. Each of you knows the specific part you played:

- In memory of Dr. Sally Schindele of Pediatric Gastroenterology of Idaho. May your family know your dedication to children's digestive health lives on in Parker and all the families touched by our story. You believed in me as a mother and without your willingness to seek out a diagnosis, we may not be where we are today.
- Thank you to the many other pediatric specialists at St. Luke's Children Hospital and Family Practice Medical Center in Boise, Idaho who willingly tested Parker for various diseases and disorders and who also heeded my mother's instinct until we found answers.
- Mary Slawson of CSIDinfo.com, your experience and knowledge provided me with the boundaries and the determination needed to make this resource both safe and practical. Though our approaches differ in many ways, I could never have completed this project without

your willingness to participate in editing my original draft back in 2008.

- Dr. Mike and Cindy Schmillen of Mountain Family Wellness Klinic in Nampa, Idaho. Your perspectives on holistic health combined with your belief in God's ultimate design for the human body will always be priceless. You helped me to bring balance and healing to Parker's sick and suffering body and for that I will always be indebted.

- Elora, you are the light of my life, my princess and my constant source of pride. I know the road has not been easy and will remain a challenge for you regarding your dietary limitations. I started this book in order to give you a place to start as you entered adulthood. I am sorry it is a little late in the making, but I am sure you will get a lot of use out if it from this point on!

- Tayler, you are my joy and my break from the storm. Your unique perspective on life constantly shows me how to look at things differently. I can't recall a single complaint from you as I shoved recipe after recipe before you. You will eat anything! You are also the first to tell me when something tastes good.

- Dawson, one day I will learn to keep our home stocked up with coconut macaroons! Your strong and gentle spirit will surely lead your own family one day in truth, both spiritually and physically.

- Jared, I just know one day you will be running your own restaurant with a special sugar and starch-free menu section. Thank you for cooking with me on many occasions and for eating many foods you would rather avoid. I can't wait to see how you take my simple recipes and turn them into famous masterpieces!

- Parker, you will never know what a blessing you are to everyone you meet! You are truly a miracle child. God has amazing plans for your life. Your encouraging hand on my shoulder as I type, your hug around my leg as I cook and your compassion for others is more than I can bear at times. This book is only a small part of my dedication to help you to live a long, healthy and happy life in order to fulfill your ultimate calling.

- To my mother, Christina Ivazes, for instilling in me the ability to give my children nothing less than the best in health and nutrition. Without the foundation you gave me from the time I was a small child, I would have not known where to begin!
- To my father, Phil Pinkerton and his wife, Nadia for their unending encouragement. Though our visits are few and far between, you have always encouraged me to do my best and to use my talents wisely.
- I will be eternally grateful to my spiritual shepherds Pastor Wayne, Pastor Amy and Pastor Scott; to my spiritual parents, Ken and Cindy, Lee and Gloria, Dan and Carolyn, Dan and Joyce, Ron and Tammy, and many others.
- To my spiritual brothers and sisters - I know I will miss someone if I try to list you all here but you know who you are - you have believed in me and encouraged me more than you know. I could never express my gratitude sufficiently with words alone.
- Next, I am thankful to my sisters, Sara, Amber, and Crystal; and to my best friends for life Tara and Tanya, I could not do life without you! Your unending support and interest in the lives of me and my husband and our children, your tenacity and your perspectives ground me and give me focus always.
- In addition to dedicating this book to you, I must also express thanks to the many CSID parents who have given me words of support, tried my recipes, provided feedback and more.
- Finally, I thank my husband, Mike for his unconditional love, his willingness to work hard to finance the many aspects required for me to complete this book, and for eating many foods and meals he would never normally eat. Honey, I know it has not been easy, but it has been worth it. Your support has not only allowed me to feed our own family better, but is now reaching the world to help countless other families! I love you!

Introduction

I have created *A Place to Start Without Sugar or Starch* as a way to share all I have learned with parents, caregivers, dietitians and doctors in order to give them a place to begin managing the CSID diet with some level of confidence.

CSID (Congenital Sucrase Isomaltase Deficiency) is a genetic digestive disorder that affects two of my children, me and an estimated undiagnosed and suffering 1 million Americans. More limiting than Celiac disease, the dietary restrictions of CSID expand far beyond the scope of simply eliminating gluten. Initial elimination of all starches and sugars is essential, followed by slowly adding easy to digest carbohydrates until tolerance levels are determined.

For parents of young children and infants, this process can be overwhelming and frustrating. After all, how does a young child grow with the absence of carbohydrates from their diet? Aside from descriptions of its cause via online medical websites and professional journals largely inaccessible to the public there is not a single resource published regarding the management of the CSID diet. Understanding the cause of CSID hardly addresses the main concern of most parents I come in contact with.

What we all want and need to know is what do we feed our child and how do we repair the months or years of damage done by the indigested food wreaking havoc within their bodies?

The number of children and adults diagnosed with CSID has multiplied dramatically over the past several years. At the time of Parker's diagnosis in 2005, a little over 400 children and adults had been diagnosed with CSID in the entire world. As of the date of this publication, the latest numbers reported on CSIDinfo.com claim worldwide diagnosis is at 7512!

These numbers could just be breaking the ice. According to information recently shared with me by Parker's gastroenterologist, studies have now indicated thousands of cases of chronic infant and childhood diarrhea are now thought to be CSID!

During the frustrating journey to discover the foods and supplements needed to bring my son to good health, I saw a grave need to share all I had learned with other moms. Every time I conducted an internet search for CSID and related terms in hopes for answers, I came across the same websites which seemed to be directed toward doctors and dietitians more than to parents.

Most of them simply sum up the cause of CSID and that Sucraid (an enzyme therapy available by prescription only) is needed to help in digesting sucrose. In addition, my online searching often led me to numerous queries from dietitians and doctors who had patients with a diagnosis but no real understanding of how to direct them in eating the appropriate foods.

Today, I am regularly contacted by parents who come across my blog (www.csidrecipes.com) or Facebook page asking about solutions as to where to begin in feeding their child. The need for a book about CSID is undeniable. Parents of recently and long-term CSID diagnosed children are frustrated and discouraged at the limited information available online and in published form.

Digestive books don't mention it. Cookbooks on sugar-free and gluten-free recipes don't discuss it. Doctors don't and sometimes won't test for it in many cases. Most dietitians know nothing about it. In my research I have found that even most GI medical books don't even reference the disorder at all!

Where does that leave the over seven thousand people with a CSID diagnosis? Other parents and adults experienced with managing CSID are their only hope for a step in the right direction.

With many years of research, trial, error and a lifetime of nutrition and holistic digestive health knowledge and practice, I now consider it my duty to share all I have learned from a practical approach. Is managing and mastering the CSID diet easy? Never. I fail almost daily at reaching the high standards I set forth in this book.

However, with knowledge comes power and I firmly believe that any child with a parent determined to gain an understanding of the optimal way to care for them will be far better off for life. Because of all I now know about CSID and digestive health through diet, it is easier to set dietary limits for my family and our recovery time after "giving in" to taboo foods is far shorter than any medical reports I have read.

My countless hours of researching digestion and finding the best food combinations and digestive supplements have revealed that the CSID diet can also benefit those with Celiac disease, Crohn's, colitis, diabetes and even fibromyalgia.

The continual theme throughout this book is to assist parents in creating a lifestyle of providing healing foods and some of the healthiest foods on the planet. It can be summed up with this phrase:

Add what helps and remove what harms.

This is not a quick-fix or a list of recipes designed to mimic the already unhealthy American, fast-food diet. Although I feel I have a realistic approach, my philosophy is that if I am going to take the time to make a meal for my family, using the healthiest, best ingredients is my only option. Otherwise, I may as well just pop a pre-packaged meal in the oven or go through the drive-through.

Preface: My CSID Story

Grab a chair and find a few minutes of quiet in order to read my story in the next few pages. Though the journey hasn't been perfect, and I am still learning, learning my story is an important part in understanding how this book you hold came to be. It is nothing less than a labor of love and an extension of the grace, guidance and favor God has shown me since the day I became a mother.

OUR PERSONAL STORY
1994

I was a new mom and wife and as young as I was (18)—I knew I wanted the best for my daughter. I planned to breastfeed Elora and make all of her food from scratch. I even intended on using cloth diapers. I had the desire to 'parent naturally' in every sense of the word. But, I was young, and with the many other challenges in my life, I found it difficult to follow through.

When Elora started formula at three months old, she began having increased and loose bowel movements and had several "yeast rashes". Eventually her doctor put her on soy formula, thinking she was reacting to the milk protein. Though it didn't completely clear up her symptoms, her diaper rashes became fewer and far between and we assumed she had a milk allergy.

This seemed to be confirmed one night, when she was about ten months old. We had run out of formula and I gave her a small bottle of milk. I remember her little belly distended out and her standing in her crib screaming and crying for what seemed like hours. I knew she was in pain, but I didn't know how to fix it.

Looking back, I am not so sure it was the milk that had been the main culprit. The milk probably just intensified whatever I had served her for dinner as it had likely contained high levels of starches and natural sugars.

We continued using the soy formula until she was about 18 months old and then she seemed to do fine with cow's milk. Though her belly bulged out in front of her skinny legs, the doctors never aired the slightest concern about her health or digestion. She continued to have runny bowel movements and diaper rashes. Doctors and family convinced me this was normal, and that there was little I could do about her reoccurring yeast infections aside from frequent diaper changes.

She also wet her bed until she was nine years old and had many incidents of soiling herself through her early elementary years. As young parents, we assumed she just wasn't paying attention to her body's signals that she had to use the bathroom. Later, we realized she may not have been able to control herself.

1995

Our second daughter was born a healthy 7 pounds, 4 ounces. Aside from having reflux and drenching several burp rags per day, Tayler was a chubby, happy baby. I attributed her reflux to having swallowed meconium prior to birth which required her stomach to be pumped. She also had strange, light-colored bowel movements as an infant, even while breastfeeding.

Tayler also began formula at around three months of age. The only way she could eat without discomfort was by lying on her stomach, a difficult feat to accomplish while nursing!

Today I am aware that reflux and pale-colored bowel movements are also indicators that she is a carrier of the CSID mutation. Though starch and sugar do not seem to bother her, we are pretty sure she is lactose intolerant.

1998

Pregnant with baby number three, we settled into a small house across the street from the elementary school. Elora would be starting kindergarten that year and all seemed fine amidst the normal challenges of raising two daughters on a construction worker's income.

That year, however, I remember Elora getting sick a lot. For about four months, she would be either vomiting or having diarrhea or both. When I took her into the doctor, he just told me that the stomach flu was going around. When she had bellyaches at school, we thought it was from nerves about the new baby and the fact her daddy worked out of town for the last three months of my pregnancy.

1999

We were blessed with a little boy, and I was finally able to successfully breastfeed for ten months. But when Dawson was a few months old, Elora came down with the same 'stomach-flu-like' symptoms. We had since moved for job-related reasons and I expressed a concern to her new pediatrician about her reoccurring symptoms. He had her and Tayler tested for parasites.

When the results came back positive, I was a little confused. How come she wasn't showing any more serious symptoms considering her first bouts of vomiting had begun a year and half earlier? I never got an answer.

We moved to Idaho later that year so that my husband could start his own business. In addition to wanting to raise our kids away from the hectic and expensive lifestyle of living in Southern California, it would be easier for me to eventually stay at home permanently with our children.

Though Dawson was a very happy baby, he also suffered from horrible diaper rashes and rashes around his mouth. As he got older, I began to notice whenever he drank fruit punch or ate too much candy, his cheeks would get flushed and his lips and outside of his mouth would get irritated. He has not been tested for CSID, but I am sure he has more intolerance for high levels of sugars and starches than he cares to admit.

2001

Void of the many struggles we faced settling into Idaho, we decided to stay in the family friendly community of the Treasure Valley and the capital of Boise. My husband's business had become sufficient enough for me to quit work. Three months after I became an official stay-at-home mom, I was pregnant again! As new Christians, we grew a lot in our faith that year, believing God would provide for my husband's business, give us discernment for an unruly neighbor, and to help us accept all the responsibilities and blessings that came with our growing family.

At my 20-week check-up and ultrasound, a birth defect was discovered along with the news we would be having another boy. Our fourth child had an abnormal kidney, and would possibly need surgery. This was the first time we would be facing a diagnosed health concern in one of our children, and our faith began to play a bigger part than ever in our lives. Though this may seem unrelated to the other children's digestive issues, I must note that I am aware of at least two other mothers who have children with CSID with a sibling with kidney problems. This is an odd, yet interesting coincidence to say the least.

2002

After my first induced labor and epidural, our fourth child, Jared, was born seemingly healthy and strong. His doctor put him on preventative antibiotics to avoid infection as he carefully monitored his kidney. Jared had several tests and procedures throughout the year, introducing me to hospital procedures and the various children's departments at the hospital.

Although Jared seems to be the only one of our children without obvious digestive sensitivities, the process I went through during his tests and hospital stays prepared me for what I would eventually experience with Parker, our fifth child, and our long struggle which eventually led to Parker's CSID diagnosis.

2003

When Jared was a year-old he had a severe kidney infection and was hospitalized for five days. Upon consultation with his urologist, we agreed surgery was now a necessary step in ensuring Jared's long-term health. By the time we had scheduled the surgery in April, I was already pregnant again. Although this new pregnancy planted new found fears in both my husband and I regarding provision for our family's needs, I discovered a new level of faith while I watched Jared sleeping in the hospital room after his surgery.

What was supposed to be a precautionary over-night stay post-surgery, turned into another five days. Jared's kidney had not responded well to the surgery and the trauma had caused his entire digestive system to seize up. I couldn't even hold him as his belly filled with air and even the slightest movement caused him to scream out in pain. He would have to undergo another procedure immediately. A nephrostomy tube had to be inserted into his kidney from the outside of his lower back. This would drain the fluid collecting in his kidney until the swelling went down enough to assess the next step to take to repair his kidney permanently.

I clearly remember standing by his hospital crib late that evening, as he slept through the screams of the child in the adjacent room. I had started praying for strength to get through the night and whatever challenges caring for him would entail over the next weeks or months.

Although it wasn't an audible voice, in my mind, I clearly heard the words: *I am preparing you for something else.*

At the time I didn't know if that 'something else' had to do with Jared, but I held onto those words over the next several months. After a half-a-dozen additional procedures, Jared's kidney finally began functioning normally by mid-October of that year; those words quickly became a distant memory.

Oddly enough, and even after constant antibiotics for nearly two years, Jared is a healthy ten-year-old boy. I often tease him that although he is the pickiest eater of all his siblings, he is very lucky that he can eat virtually anything without suffering from a tummy ache!

2004

After experiencing insomnia and extreme pelvic pain the last several weeks of my pregnancy, I was induced during the first week of March. Though the beginning of my labor was long, as soon as the epidural kicked in, I was ready to give birth to our fifth child.

Parker James was born 6 pounds, 10 ounces and 18 ½ inches long. Though he was smaller than the average seven pounds, twenty inches of my other children, he appeared a healthy newborn.

However, his blood sugar levels dropped below normal before we were discharged and I was encouraged to nurse him as often as possible. He was having difficulty latching on, and kept falling asleep before my milk let down. He also had excess mucus which seemed to choke him several times during each feeding.

I took him to the hospital lactation consultant when he was around one week old to determine if a different approach was needed. Aside from finding different positions to make latching on easier, there was not much more I could do. I started pumping after each feeding to ensure an adequate milk supply. Though he wasn't growing as rapidly as my other children, he gained about ½ ounce a day for the first several months. I was in no hurry to introduce solid foods, and did what I could to nourish myself enough to keep up with his frequent feedings.

Then, when he was about six months old, he started having breath-holding spells—a very scary, seizure-like episode where instead of crying, he would just turn gray, arch back and pass out. Any concerns the doctors or myself had about him not growing were put on the back burner. He was evaluated by a neurologist and a gastroenterologist to determine if there was a physical explanation for his spells.

Normally, children don't start breath-holding until they are two years old. Parker wasn't old enough to self-induce a tantrum, and my instincts told me there was something else going on. We could only find out what that was by exhausting all other possibilities. After an eeg, ekg and other tests over two hospital stays, he was found to have reflux and was put on the antacid Prevacid.

I was also giving him cups of diluted pear juice and aloe vera, in an attempt to sooth any discomfort from the spells. (Of course, now I realize pear juice contains high levels of sucrose and was probably exacerbating his symptoms!)

At the same time Parker had also developed a mild, unexplained rash on his cheeks. When I pointed this out to the doctors, they didn't seem too concerned. At his nine-month check-up, I asked about the rash again and noted several other oddities about Parker's physical appearance and behavior. Parker had a webbing of his second and third toes, a slight inward curve to both his small fingers, and always had a runny nose. He had also had a few unexplained episodes of vomiting without a fever; frequent, very smelly bowel movements; and often experienced night sweats. I was hoping a discussion of the combination of his symptoms would trigger some type of diagnosis.

After determining he had hardly grown in the previous 3 months, he was given a failure-to-thrive diagnosis considered unrelated to his breath-holding episodes and other symptoms. I continued to mention all of these symptoms during every doctor's appointment. Each time I was assured that all of these rarities in one child were not connected and that he would likely "grow out of them" without explanation.

Then, the day after Christmas, 2004, Parker had a severe breath-holding spell which was followed by a grand mal seizure which lasted five minutes. After being monitored over-night at the hospital, no further seizure activity was detected. Since he had been running a small fever prior to the seizure, this event was written off as isolated and unconnected to Parker's other issues.

March 2005

I, my husband, Parker's grandparents and other family members were frustrated by the lack of answers. However, we are grateful that most of the doctors and specialists who saw Parker took our concerns to heart and conducted whatever tests they could to pinpoint a diagnosis. Parker was tested for growth-hormone deficiency, Celiac disease, other food allergies, and even stayed in the hospital over his first birthday for a 24-hour eeg-ekg monitoring test.

During this five-day stay in the children's ward, he was also given his first dose of Phenobarbital (drowning in sucrose syrup no less) and immediately threw it up. Even though he was not having regular seizure activity, the doctor thought maybe the Phenobarbital would calm his nervous system enough to stop the breath-holding spells, which occurred as frequently as eight times per day.

By the next day, he had continued throwing up and began having diarrhea as well. After two more days in the hospital, a CT scan, and an evaluation of one of his soiled diapers by the lab, he was sent home. Everyone assumed he had caught a stomach virus from being in the children's ward for so long. (The fact he had eaten macaroni and cheese and birthday cake in the hospital was not considered a factor at all.) Something in the back of my mind thought that sounded familiar, as I recalled Elora's bouts of so-called stomach flu as a child, but what was I to do? The doctors really seemed to be doing all they could.

I cannot say that I was not frustrated and concerned with my son's health. I cannot say that I never doubted I had done something to cause his discomfort. However, every once in a while, after catching up on my sleep and getting a moment of quiet in our small apartment with our five children (who I was also homeschooling!), I would remember that night in the hospital with Jared.

I am preparing you for something else.

I would hold on another day, or another week, or however long I needed to face the next mountain. I learned to accept what I could not change. I kept detailed records about Parker including sleep patterns, foods, and sensitivities to the environment. I had started journaling all the food he ate, how often he nursed, and all his symptoms or odd behavior.

To protect him from breath-holding spells and seizures often induced by his rambunctious siblings, Parker became a silent and content fixture on my hip. One day, I remember working in the kitchen for about an hour when I suddenly noticed Parker watching my every move. I had been so focused on whatever I was cooking or cleaning I had literally forgotten I was holding him! Despite all that he had endured, he had such a calm and sweet spirit about him when he was in my arms.

After the hospital stay on his birthday, he was nursing every 20 minutes, and I finally gave in and fed him a bottle of formula in order to give myself time to rehydrate. He sucked it down in no time (probably due to dehydration), and though I continued to nurse him for a few more months, formula supplements soon became part of his daily diet.

The next time he saw the doctor, he had gained several ounces. This was a huge milestone as he had hardly grown in length or weight during the six months prior. Sighing with relief, we all assumed this was the answer to his failure to grow well—he just wasn't getting enough calories from my breast milk! Even though he continued to have rashes, six or more foul-smelling-bulky diapers per day, and several breath holding spells followed by minor seizures, we were all relieved that he had started growing.

By 16 months old, Parker was breastfeeding only at night. I had started giving him goat's milk, which he seemed to tolerate well. For solid foods, I was feeding him home-made brown rice, lentils, and yams (all very high in starch content but I did not know any better at that time). He also ate what the family ate for dinner from spaghetti to fried chicken to fast food. I tried to eliminate anything that seemed to cause the rash on his face to flare up, but I found it hard to determine as sometimes his siblings would also feed him without my knowledge. I had come to the conclusion that I had done all I could do, and that those words I felt God telling me were for me to learn to accept the unknown.

Then Parker's seizures started coming more frequently. He was napping up to four hours at one time on the days he experienced several breath-holding spells and seizures.

Parker had also come to a wall in his verbal and motor skills progress. Though he took his first steps at ten months, he didn't begin to fully walk until he was fourteen months old. He didn't seem interested in speaking either, and he couldn't even cry without going into a breath-holding spell. Everyone in the house had to learn to watch him carefully while anticipating his every need and want.

August 2005

I consulted his neurologist and as much as I hated the idea of Parker going on daily medication, I yielded to his suggestion to start Phenobarbital.

After just a few doses, the seizure activity stopped. Parker was up and about more often for the next several weeks, but he soon went quickly downhill.

October 2005

At the beginning of October 2005, over the course of a few days, Parker had become extremely lethargic. He couldn't seem to stay awake, and would fuss weakly when he was. His appetite decreased and he kept falling asleep. He had several yucky bowel movements, but I was so used to them by that point, I didn't think they were an indication that something else was going on.

Having little faith that any of his doctors would have a different answer for me, I sent out an email request for prayer to everyone I knew. Parker needed a miracle, and honestly, so did I! I was exhausted and didn't have the strength to face another slew of tests and hospital stays with my hurting baby.

That Thursday, Parker had a follow-up appointment with his pediatric gastroenterologist, Dr. Sally Schindele. He took his normal morning nap before his appointment, but still proceeded to fall asleep on my lap while we waiting for the doctor. When she came in and began the exam, Parker remained sleeping. This was very unusual. After all, even the most miserable 18-month old would at least protest with a small whimper in response to the ice-cold stethoscope. But he kept sleeping.

Dr. Schindele sat down and slowly began flipping through Parker's chart. I could tell she was concerned, but didn't want to alarm me. After several minutes, she asked me if I could remember why we never did a small bowel biopsy.

I shook my head in response, smiled weakly and said, "No, I don't. You have done every other test."

The only reason why I think she didn't admit Parker to the children's ward to be treated for dehydration was because of all we had already been through. If he got worse, I was to bring him to the ER. She scheduled the biopsy for the following Thursday and sent us home.

He didn't have a single wet diaper all day, but stayed awake for the rest of the afternoon, though in a daze. He only he sipped on goat's milk and pear juice three or four times and continued to refuse any solid foods.

On Friday, his appetite decreased even more and he had seven bowel movements. I weighed him and realized he had lost weight. His belly was swollen and had a grayish tint to it. He did not have the energy to move around the house, and would start fussing when he wasn't near me. He managed to drink around 10 ounces of goat's milk and some pear juice before falling asleep for the night.

On Saturday, he had a wet diaper upon waking up. This was a good sign and probably the only thing that kept me from rushing him to the ER. He didn't have a bowel movement until around noon, dissipating any thought that he was dehydrated. Though he was still very weak and falling in and out of sleep, I decided not to give him any goat milk or pear juice that day just to be safe.

Somehow, he managed to recover enough over the next few days to be well for his biopsy procedure. Though I had a thousand questions, I knew this was the last straw. If we didn't get answers this time, we would just have to find a way to care for Parker despite the unknown.

When the doctor came to tell us she was done with the procedure, she carefully sat down between my husband and me before telling us what she had found.

Again, a look of concern crossed her face as she tried to explain what she had seen during the biopsy. If we agreed, she wanted to have a CT scan done of Parker's chest before he left the hospital. His esophagus tube was extremely narrow right about the point where his aorta valve would be attached. If his aorta valve was wrapped around his esophagus, he would need heart surgery. This could explain his breath holding spells, and if his heart was working overtime due to a birth defect, his slow growth could also be explained. We would still not understand his other ailments, but it would be a start. However, we would not get the results of the CT scan until Monday.

I think that weekend tested my faith more than ever. If Parker needed heart surgery, there would be a huge risk factor involved. He could even die. Was this what God was preparing me for? I didn't know what choice I had, and I just let it all go; all the control I thought I had over Parker's well-being. I gave it all to God and told Him I would accept the diagnosis, no matter what sacrifice it entailed.

At eight am Monday morning, the phone rang. My heart fluttered and raced as I answered the phone. It was the Dr. Schindele. She immediately told me Parker's heart looked fine. I let out a huge sigh; as if I had been holding my breath for three days, and tears stung my eyes.

She could not explain what was causing the narrow opening, but nonetheless it was likely being constrained when Parker became upset. At least now we had an explanation for why he could not catch his breath on his own. The rest of the test results would take a couple of weeks to come through.

FINALLY, A DIAGNOSIS!

The week before Halloween, the final results came through.

"Parker has Congenital Sucrase-Isomaltase Deficiency." His doctor said slowly over the phone.

I grabbed a pencil and a notepad. "Spell that for me and then tell me what it means!" I could hear the relief in my voice and I think I may have even been smiling. I had no idea what Parker had, but I was too relieved to care. We finally had an answer—a diagnosis!

Oh, if I only knew! All his doctor knew about CSID was that Parker couldn't eat "table sugar" or starch. I would have to look up more information online and seek the guidance of a dietitian to help curb his diet. After a huge sigh of relief, I prepared myself for the work it would entail to finally know what to feed my son.

I felt very equipped and capable to handle this newfound challenge, even with all the other commitments in my life. I was finishing my degree online and had learned how to effectively research on the web. I immediately searched for the CSID web site the doctor had given me, registered at NORD (national organization for rare diseases), and made an appointment with a dietitian.

It didn't take long for me to realize why Parker's doctor couldn't tell me more. There were only a handful of references to CSID, and they all pretty much summed up the cause and vaguely discussed the elimination of starches and the need for Sucraid [1] to digest sugar.

I received the most information from the administrator of the CSID parent support group web site, Mary Slawson. Mary explained that because each child has a different mutation of CSID, the amount of starches and sugars each person can tolerate varies. My best option was to find a dietitian that would help me create the perfect diet to meet Parker's specific needs.

At this point, I was feeling more overwhelmed than hopeful. My hope faded even further when I found out I

---

[1] Sucraid (Sacrosidase) is an enzyme replacement therapy specifically designed for those with Congenital Sucrase Isomaltase Deficiency. It is available by prescription only. For more information see www.sucraid.net.

needed to pay cash for the dietitian because she didn't accept my son's insurance. In addition, it was a forty-minute drive to her office. However, the drive was worth it as the dietitian boosted my confidence and helped me to make a plan. I was still going to be on my own, but she gave me several pointers for food options that steered me in the right direction.

The first step was to eliminate the 2 teaspoons of the sucrose-based syrup Phenobarbital Parker was taking each day. His neurologist ordered a pill form of the medication, which we started putting in yogurt.

My notebooks came out again, and I began to chart everything Parker ate, all his symptoms, and when I gave him Sucraid. I initially thought he was in Group C, so I continue to feed him starches. After reviewing his specific enzyme levels with Mary a few weeks later, she then told me he was in Group B.

I was devastated to learn I had still been feeding Parker food he wasn't supposed to have! No more puffed rice cereal or oatmeal. I had to narrow of his food options once again. Even the slightest trace of starch in the ingredient list on a food label soon indicated that item was off the list of permissible foods. When family members or caregivers asked me what Parker could not eat, I would laugh and tell them it was probably easier for me to just tell them the eight things he could have!

In addition to the changes we were making in his diet, Parker's dad and I also weaned him off Phenobarbital. It was a hassle to get him to eat it in the yogurt, and Parker had still not made significant improvements in his speech and motor skills.

Within two days of removing Phenobarbital, Parker began talking! At this point, I had removed all known sugars and starches from his diet. Do you think it is a coincidence that he never had another seizure? This confirmed what I had thought all along—that Parker's seizures did have something to do with his failure to thrive and his inability to digest food!

At first, however, Parker still did not appear to tolerate many of the foods he supposedly could digest. Rashes would come and go, and no matter how little fruit I gave him with Sucraid, he still had diarrhea. With the approval of his dietitian, I also started feeding him small amounts of almond flour-based goods such as bread and pancakes.

After experimenting with various foods and supplements, my first notes showing Parker was symptom free were in March of 2006, over four months following his diagnosis. However, on the same day I also increased his serving of pears and applesauce which resulted in several loose BMs, despite having given him Sucraid. A short time later, I decided to stop Sucraid since Parker seemed to only tolerate a few ounces of sucrose containing foods. I realized determining which foods he could tolerate without Sucraid was an important next step.

The next several months, Parker's diet was very restricted as I focused on feeding him vegetables, meat proteins, and dairy products. I did not give him any food that I knew contained any forms of sucrose or starches (including soy flakes). By January, 2007, I was ready to introduce Sucraid again.

Shortly afterwards, Parker began developing a rash on his face. Since I had not changed a whole lot in his diet, and since he was not having diarrhea, I was unsure at what was causing it. I assumed one of his sisters had given him something and that the rash would clear up.

Then my husband asked if I had checked the label on the tuna recently. As soon as he said it, I knew. I had failed to double check the ingredient label on the tuna for weeks. After all, it was just tuna in water so what could change? Sure enough, the manufacturer had started adding soy flakes! Within a few days of treating his rash with ointment and removing the tuna and other canned fish we had been feeding him that had also begun adding soy flakes, his rash cleared up.

FROM SURVIVING TO THRIVING
May 2007

During a church barbeque where the Christian Motorcycle association was serving hamburgers, one of them starting asking about Parker after I had asked if the hamburgers were 100% beef. Her husband had suffered from digestive problems and had started seeing an alternative medicine doctor. On Monday, I called to make an appointment. I was not sure what they could do for Parker, but I knew his health could still improve.

It is only a miracle that they had an opening for testing that Thursday and we just happened to have additional money available to cover the costs. The testing they did was non-invasive and peaceful compared to the hospital procedures he had experienced. They measure the stress levels of all his vital organs in a test called a Thermography, and took saliva and urine samples to measure his pH and salt levels.

Their diagnosis: Parker's internal organs; especially his intestines and stomach, were still highly stressed, despite having removed troubling foods from his diet.

Though it took a few minutes to sink in, and though I came close to tears thinking how Parker still was not as healthy as he could be; I had to be grateful that I was getting *answers* PLUS *solutions* this time around. This doctor had a plan and she believed Parker could achieve maximum health and well-being to his body if we worked together to assist him. The plan included various supplements and digestive support therapy, along with a few adjustments to his current diet.

October 2008

By this time, my oldest daughter, Elora was fourteen. The previous July she had been in a severe car accident. Weeks of bed rest and medication had added to my role as caregiver and nurse for her as well as for Parker. After her initial recovery, her older symptoms of digestion problems surfaced once again. After a severe bout of stomach cramping and indigestion, we finally had her seen by our pediatric GI for testing.

She had eaten an excess of pizza and pasta over the weekend. Her belly bloated out and she had sharp pains all around her upper back and chest. She told me she wanted to know if she had CSID. I had a hunch she would and we all knew she would be giving up her favorite foods include pizza and pasta, if the results were positive!

Sure enough, three years almost to the day after Parker's diagnosis, Elora's results were positive as well. Realizing the dilemma in re-teaching my 14-year-old how to eat and make choices for herself, I submitted to the fact it was finally time I wrote a book about all I had learned.

2012

Having children with CSID is about more than a quick fix for finding the meals for the day. It has become a lifestyle for our whole family in both understanding and in practice.

My hope in compiling what I have learned into a single reference guide is that parents who read this book will be able to focus their efforts in caring for their child. You don't have to spend hours on the internet, in book stores or the library, trying to figure out what you can eat.

You hold in your hands a comprehensive starting place to help you care for you or your child's dietary needs now. It will take time getting used to, sacrifice, adjusting your budget, and a few long grocery-shopping adventures. In the end, your happy, healthy child, will be worth it!

In the four years since I have started this book project, there have been many challenges and triumphs. I have had to change my approach and apply certain measures to protect myself and those who may flip directly to my recipes without fully understanding that their child's digestive needs are unique.

I have struggled with staying consistent in fe family and have discovered that I personally feel mu when sticking with the foods and recipes outlinec book. Educating my own children about wise food ch ⌐ ⌐ is one of my main priorities as one day they have a chance of having children with CSID themselves. Money and time constraints have not always made it possible to provide the ideal diet. However, I take much comfort in knowing how to steer us all back on a path of healthy eating, when taking that path is possible.

On a positive and encouraging note, Parker and Elora now fall under Group C and are able to tolerate some starch. Although we do include the occasional brown rice or gluten-free pasta dish in our personal diet, these foods are not tolerated by some CSID groups and are excluded from this book. I have learned that these foods are still not beneficial in excess. From my research and personal experience, avoiding starchy vegetables such as potatoes and corn as well as grains such as wheat, oats, barley and rice produce fewer digestive problems in the long-term.

As the title suggests, what I offer here is simply *a place to start* and the best way I have come to learn how to feed my own family. May you glean what meets the current needs of your family and find inspiration to begin your own personal journey of discovering additional foods and recipes in the months and years to come.

2016

Since the printing of the first edition, my children have gone through various struggles. Parker acquired numerous food allergies shortly after publishing when his school failed to ensure he was taking his enzymes with meals. There were also some undetermined environmental factors, which I believe were associated with the apartment complex where we lived as well as the school building.

Thankfully, about that time I was beginning to learn more about how the Paleo diet could benefit our family. I obtained a copy of Diane Sanfilippo's book *Practical Paleo* and it forever changed my outlook on what certain foods could do to an already compromised digestive system. Instead of revising the recipes in this book, however, I've decided to point you toward her book as a key reference and resource in understanding digestion and pinpointing possible problem foods specific to your situation.

Although I wanted to do a thorough revise of this book, I realize there are parents and adults out there in need of the basic information now. My blog goes into more details about the solutions and strategies I used to help Parker recover from a year-long eczema flare-up. And I'm happy to report as of publication he has overcome all his food allergies except for shrimp.

Additionally, my oldest son, Dawson, has a recent diagnosis of Celiac Disease. His GI doesn't think it's related to CSID, but since he's a sibling, it's possible an illness he had in elementary school could have "turned on" the celiac response. So, we are now dealing with a gluten-allergy in addition to CSID limitations.

I highly encourage you to subscribe to my blog at www.csidrecipes.com for updates on my family and links to information I discover in my own CSID journey.

Note about Sucraid: Our family does not currently use Sucraid for various reasons. As a result, I have removed reference to its use in the recipe section, though foods that contain natural sucrose levels are noted to the best of my knowledge.

If you would like more information about Sucraid, see the reference section for links.

PART 1 - PROBLEMS AND CAUSES

"God created the law of free will, and God created the law of cause and effect. And he himself will not violate the law. We need to be thinking less in terms of what God did and more in terms of whether or not we are following those laws."
Marianne Williamson

1 - Food Intolerance Causes and Symptoms

This Book Is Not About Food Allergies

Food allergies are a separate and often more serious issue caused by an immediate response from the immune system. This book does not cover food allergies for two reasons. For one, food allergies are easier to diagnose thus the prevalence of positive diagnosis and books on the subject.

Secondly, due to the seriousness of food allergies I cannot address both food allergies and food intolerance at the same time. Since the original printing, Parker developed food allergies to wheat, milk, egg whites, and shrimp along with too many environmental allergies to note here. After over 2 years of additional diet modifications and the inclusion of digestive supplements, his most recent allergy tests reveal he is now only allergic to shrimp! The reasons he acquired and then recovered from most of the food allergies are all conjecture, so I have decided not to address specific food allergies at this time.

Any reference to food allergies in this book is only to call attention to the differences in allergy and intolerance and is not meant to diagnose or cure children with food allergies.

Food Intolerance

Food intolerance may take days or weeks to surface and may only occur after significant accumulation of the offending food. Food intolerance is in its essence the inability to digest a specific food, or an overabundance of a specific food. Lactose is the most common culprit of food intolerance.

There are various symptoms associated with food intolerance in infants ranging from diaper rash to failure to thrive, dehydration, or seizures. In addition, the more common symptoms associated with food intolerance such as gas, bloating and indigestion are experienced at all ages. Many of the symptoms are similar regardless of the type of food a person is having trouble with, as symptoms only reveal that the body is struggling either internally or externally.

same symptoms can also be related to environmental _____ such as common household cleaners.

Knowing It's Food Is the Hardest Part

Many early signs of food intolerance, such as diaper rash, vomiting or diarrhea are often overlooked. Parents and doctors can easily ignore these symptoms, assuming they were caused by infrequent diaper changes or a stomach virus. I can recall a conversation with one parent years ago in which they were told that any time a child starts a new food, diarrhea was normal and that over time their body would adjust!

So when do we, as parents, know it is food that is causing the problem? Though there is no easy answer, chronic (or ongoing) verses acute (isolated) is a general rule of thumb. A good starting place is to understand what can cause food intolerance to begin with. Then we can look at some of the common and not so common problem foods. If altering the diet through eliminating these foods also eliminates or decreases symptoms, you will also have a place to start regarding which foods to avoid.

First, here is a little background as to how I discovered many of the foundational premises regarding digestive health.

Understanding the Specific Carbohydrate Diet™ in Light of CSID

The day my eyes truly opened to the havoc happening inside my son's body was the day I read *Breaking the Vicious Cycle* by Elaine Gottschall at the recommendation of my son's dietitian. Elaine goes into great detail regarding the consequences undigested carbohydrates have in the gut. You will recognize descriptions of these consequences as the symptoms our children experienced before and even after their CSID diagnosis. Though she does not mention CSID by name, she mentions the prevalence of chronic infant diarrhea and that the possible cause could be limited enzymes to digest carbohydrates.

Though all SCD "legal foods" do not match up with CSID foods, many of my recipes resulted from cross-referencing recipes containing ingredients considered "legal" for the

Specific Carbohydrate Diet (SCD) with the food lists provided on the www.csidinfo.com website. I encourage you to get your own copy of *Breaking the Vicious Cycle* to better understand why, regardless of starch content; I do not include grains in the CSID diet. The SCD diet calls for almond flour as a grain substitute because it does not encourage the growth of harmful bacteria that thrive from the carbohydrates in grains and sugars. In addition, it's much easier to digest than other nut flours, gluten-free or grain-based flours.

To clarify, not all of the recipes in this book are SCD legal, primarily since I do use ingredients containing lactose. In addition, not all SCD legal foods are appropriate for all CSID groups. For example, pumpkin, walnuts, and some of the 'legal' fruits contain too much starch or sugar to be tolerable for those with the lowest levels of maltase enzymes, or for use without Sucraid. The science behind the SCD diet is also decades old and does not account for recent discoveries of digestive related disease or disorders such as CSID. Please keep this in mind if you choose to acquire any of the many recipe books available which contain recipes designed around the Specific Carbohydrate Diet.

Causes of Food Intolerance

Two main causes of food intolerance are congenital and trauma induced intolerance.

Congenital Food Intolerance

Recent research indicates some children are born with genetic abnormalities that result in allergies, food intolerance, and/or enzyme deficiencies. This means a child is born with less than the normal amounts of enzymes to digest a particular food. Most of the research suggests this comes from inheriting specific DNA mutations from both parents. For those with CSID, their families come from England, Australia, New Zealand, Ireland, Germany, Baltic States, Scandinavia, Eastern Europe, Russia (St. Petersburg area), Iceland, Greenland, Eskimo populations in Alaska and Canada, Turkey and areas around the Black Sea. Often both the mother's and father's side of the family heritage can be traced back to the Vikings[2]. This is similar to the genetic connection between lactose intolerance and those with Asian, Indian, and Hispanic lineage.

If the child has genetically triggered food intolerance, initial symptoms will begin to appear shortly after solid foods are introduced. However, if the child is breastfed, this can be more difficult to determine since the current research is unclear as to how the child responds to food passed from the mother through the breast milk. Additionally, there is now conclusive evidence that the oligosaccharides found in breast milk protect against diarrhea in breastfed infants.[3]

In retrospect, I know for certain my son displayed problems with his digestion from birth, and though he was exclusively breastfed for nearly nine months, he was already showing signs of slow growth, frequent bowel movements, and unexplained rashes. One reason for these symptoms could be that he was getting enough sucrose and starch through my breast milk to cause his digestive system problems. This makes sense, given we now know he was born with CSID, and the inability to digest normal amounts of sucrose and starch.

Trauma Induced Intolerance
Another known cause agreed upon among experts in digestive enzyme deficiencies occurs when there has been a trauma to the digestive system. This can happen after short or long term use of antibiotics, a bacterial infection that resulted in excess vomiting and diarrhea, and even car accidents. In addition, it is possible people born with an enzyme deficiency do not display regular symptoms until a trauma kicks it into action.

This occurred with my oldest daughter, who had some CSID symptoms prior to age five, but then after being in a car accident at age 15, began presenting more severe symptoms and soon after tested positive for CSID.

If there is not a genetic disorder, a person's enzymes will return normal after a short period of avoiding the problem

---

[2] www.csidinfo.com/Introduction

[3] The Journal of Pediatrics. Volume 145, Issue 3 , Pages 297-303, September 2004

food(s). For others, a longer-term, limited diet, often eliminating milk products (since the lactase enzyme is often affected during digestive stress), is needed to allow the body sufficient time to recover.

There is the rare occasion, where permanent damage takes place, and the body can no longer produce the proper levels of enzymes. This is the case in those with trauma-induced intolerance. The most common enzymes affected are those made to digest disaccharides or those that break down lactose, sucrose, and maltose. The result is permanent lactose intolerance, Disaccharide Deficiency, Fructose Intolerance, Sucrase-Isomaltase Deficiency, or a combination of them.

Lactose Intolerance & CSID

Even after removing the sugars and starches from his diet, my son still suffered from breath-holding spells and failure to thrive. I had increased his animal protein intake, especially cheese, to overcompensate for the other foods I had eliminated. A visit to his homeopath revealed an inappropriate protein/carbohydrate ratio, causing secondary symptoms related to liver and kidney stress.

There was a period of time where I removed all dairy products with the exception of homemade yogurt. When Parker began to thrive as a result, I realized that it was possible he had been experiencing temporary lactose intolerance as a result of his damaged digestion system. It wasn't until I found a balance in his intake of protein/vegetables/dairy along with the addition of digestive-aid supplements that the other symptoms eventually ceased.

In total, he went approximately 18 months without milk or cheese products. Now, my son is able to digest dairy products without a hitch. But it took some time for his body to recover. He experienced more growth during this time than at any other time in his life. This is proof enough to me that dairy products are not always the best source of nutrients for a child struggling to thrive due to malabsorption and digestive stress.

From the less serious issue of isolated lactose intolerance to the life threatening problems associated with extreme cases CSID in infants, understanding the large array of symptoms is vital to pinpointing food sensitivity in a child early on. Please note some of these symptoms also mimic those of Celiac disease, an allergy to gluten.

Primary Symptoms of Food Intolerance
These symptoms can begin to occur minutes after eating, as with lactose intolerance, or several days as with CSID. Tracking even rare occurrences of these symptoms over time can help determine if they are related to specific food intolerance.

Note: "Symptoms" referenced throughout this book include any combination of those listed here. These symptoms should not be present for a minimum of three weeks before proceeding to advanced phases of the Induction Diet.

- stomach pain
- bloating or distention of the stomach
- excessive gas
- cramping in large intestine
- diarrhea
- constipation
- diaper rash (fermented odor)
- vomiting without a fever
- body or facial rashes
- irritability
- restlessness
- difficulty sleeping
- eczema
- frequent, smelly, acidic and/or oily bowel movements
- frequent yeast infections or yeast rashes
- failure to thrive
- irritable bowel syndrome
- excessive fussing and whining

The Following Are Not Symptoms of CSID, But May Also Be Digestive-Tract Related
Sometimes the type of food causing the problem is misinterpreted and the child or adult just accepts these

secondary symptoms as normal even after eliminating what they believe is the problem food.

Therefore, if the issue is lactose intolerance and even after removing dairy, there are still secondary symptoms, please urge your doctor to conduct further tests. If this doesn't work, begin with an induction diet as suggested in this book and see if symptoms begin to improve.

- headaches
- developmental delays
- behavior problems (autism, ADHD, etc.)
- difficulty focusing
- hay fever
- seizures
- breath-holding spells
- excessive sweating
- excess ear wax
- colic
- flu-like symptoms without a fever
- rectal bleeding or blood in stool
- frequent urinary tract infections

Preventing Initial Problems in Infants
Because there is substantial evidence showing that food allergies and intolerance are genetic, the best preventive measure parent is to delay the introduction of solid foods while exclusively breastfeeding for the first six months. Traditional first foods such as cereals can also be replaced with easier to digest foods such as bananas, avocado, and homemade yogurt.

Many packaged and processed foods, including commercially prepared infant foods, may contain unlisted ingredients. Ideally, avoid these foods until you are certain food intolerance is not a factor. See chapter 7 for more details on the importance of breastfeeding and digestive health and first foods for infants who may have food intolerance.

Preventing Long-Term Problems
If a child is born with the inability to digest sugar and starch; the condition is irreversible. Though some reports suggest CSID group B may be able to tolerate some starch after the

age of four, dietary restrictions will have to be in place for life to avoid additional ailments or digestive disease.

Health problems can occur over time and have been known to occur in relatives of positively diagnosed children. These issues can manifest if sugar (eaten without Sucraid) or starches remain in the diet at higher than tolerable levels. These problems may include:

- colon cancer
- Crohn's disease
- death by dehydration (especially in underweight and malnourished infants and toddlers)
- diverticulitis
- malabsorption/weight loss
- other digestive diseases

Though the idea of removing all foods containing sugar and starch seems exhausting and near impossible, the sooner you can learn to make needed changes, the better the chances of living a healthy and full life.

2 - Sources of Starch and Sucrose in Foods

I'm providing this chapter as a quick reference list in order to familiarize you with the various ingredients and form of sugar and starch in foods. Using this list as a reference, begin eliminating these foods and ingredients from your pantry shelves and your normal shopping list. The less of these foods you have available, the faster you and your family will become accustomed to eating CSID appropriate foods. Even if household members can tolerate these foods, exchanging them may also be needed to adjust your grocery budget.

Sources of Starch in Foods

Avoid all pre-packaged breads, cereals, crackers, chips, flour, pasta or food marked "Gluten-Free". All of these foods contain starch levels too high for groups A and B and for the initial phase of the diet which requires elimination of all harmful forms of carbohydrates. Commercially sold 'gluten-free' products contain potato, corn, tapioca, garbanzo beans, or soy. ALL of these have high levels of starches and/or carbohydrates that encourage fermentation in the gut. Once starch level tolerance is established, these foods may be consumed in limited, occasional quantities.

See Chapter 8 regarding carbohydrate essentials, the starch tolerance test and a more detailed look at the role proper carbohydrates play in the CSID diet.

Foods made from or containing starch

- baked goods (all contain flours and sugars)
- ~~beans except green beans, yellow wax, lima (butter)~~
- butternut squash, pumpkin
- corn
- corn starch, any ingredient containing 'corn'
- corn syrup
- farina (cream of wheat)
- garlic

- legumes (lentils, etc.)
- maltodextrin
- modified food starch
- oatmeal
- peas (green, split)
- potato flour, any ingredient containing 'potato'
- quinoa
- rice flour, any ingredient containing 'rice'
- soy flour, soy beans
- Splenda (sucralose)
- sun dried tomatoes
- tapioca starch or flour
- tortillas, tortilla chips
- wheat flour
- white flour
- yams

Sources of Sugar (Sucrose) in Foods
With the occasional exception, do your best to avoid or minimize these foods, even with access to Sucraid or other enzymes. Allowing an excess of refined sugars only increases the desire for sweets and offers very little (if any) nutritional benefits.

- brown sugar
- cane juice
- confectioner's sugar (powdered sugar)
- Karo syrup
- maple syrup
- molasses
- pancake syrup
- raw sugar (turbinado)
- sugar cane
- palm/coconut sugar (from coconut nectar)

(See chapter 3, *Choosing the Best Sugar Substitute* for more details.)

Food That May Require Enzymes for Sucrose Digestion

Almost any prepared or pre-packaged food contains sugar. Dressings, sauces, breads, jams, jellies, cereals, cookies, candies, pies, fruit drinks, soda, f. milk, flavored yogurt and most canned goods contain ͟c form of sugar as either a sweetener or a preservative. If there is at least

The following list includes fruits with more than 0.9 grams of naturally occurring sucrose per 100 grams. **Sucraid** or a digestive enzyme blend containing **invertase** may need to be used with some of these. Consult a health practitioner or dietitian before adding these foods.

See Chapter 5, The Induction Diet, for instructions on introducing foods containing sucrose. See Chapter 8, Essential Carbohydrates for an overview of the importance of including digestive enzymes for sugars and starches for obtaining an adequate amount of carbohydrates.

- apples
- banana (ripe with brown spots)
- blackberries
- cantaloupe
- dried apricots
- dried peach (not recommended at all)
- gooseberries
- grapefruit
- honeydew melon
- kiwi
- mandarin
- nectarine
- orange juice, oranges
- passion fruit
- peach
- pears
- pineapple
- plum
- raspberries
- strawberries
- tangelo
- watermelon

3 - Choosing the Best Sugar Substitute

I will warn you in advance, the use of sugar in the American diet frustrates me to no end. When I first started reading labels after Parker's diagnosis, I could not believe that sugar, in one form or another, was in nearly everything! To this day, I am amazed that we can live in a nation with sugar-induced health problems such as diabetes and obesity becoming the norm for preschoolers while food manufacturers profit. I strongly believe that sugars as well as refined flours have become addictive substances that are no better than drugs or alcohol.

As long as we continue to purchase foods containing these ingredients, food companies will continue to produce them. Some health-based companies are changing their ingredients to meet consumer demand. But unless consumers become better educated on what is truly "healthier," they do not hold as much power as they could in altering the types of ingredients included in prepared foods. We begin to take control of our family's diet by relearning and rethinking "normal" by excluding foods that contain sugars from the majority of our meals and snacks. Having sugar (or sweet food) with every meal is not healthy for anyone and presents serious risks for those with CSID.

In my many conversations with other CSID parents, I have found that we take a different approach regarding sugar or sugar substitutes in food. No wonder, with all the choices we have! Even with the best of intentions, we can make a wrong choice based on what we have heard or the trust that tends to occur from seeing a particular brand over and over again.

From the start, I was dead set against giving Parker any artificial sweeteners, since I knew the long term consequences would never outweigh the benefit of giving him a sweet treat. Though many people view this topic as controversial, my opinion is that my son has already suffered enough. Why would I give him a food that could bring him more harm?

The other side of this argument could be that come CSID children can only have artificial sweeteners such as aspartame. Although I can sympathize with this perspective, I also feel that this is used to justify serving diet cola, candy or gum containing aspartame or other artificial sweeteners. The bottom line is any of these foods in excess are not GOOD for ANYBODY, especially a child who is already facing lifelong challenges with making healthy food choices.

In chapter 8, I cover the issue of carbohydrate essentials and the fact that those with CSID need the carbohydrates from naturally occurring sugars in order to grow. This is especially important for those who cannot tolerate any starches. Part of this includes the use of Sucraid to assist with digestion of sucrose in foods. However, I do not condone or encourage the use of Sucraid for regular intake of sugary foods that do not serve to benefit the body in the long term. The purpose of Sucraid (in my opinion) should be to assist the child or adult with CSID in obtaining adequate sucrose-based carbohydrates from whole foods. Yes, there are exceptions such as for a birthday party or for eating at a restaurant or while traveling when there is no alternative.

I am a firm believer that knowledge equals power. My hope is that when you have the choice between two food options, you will know the best choice to make. In turn, you will be teaching your family how to make those choices one day - empowering them for a lifetime.

The ultimate goal here is teaching parents so that they can then teach their children a LIFESTYLE of eating well for total wellness:

Adding what helps and removing what harms.

I say all this as a parent who has to make daily choices regarding what is BEST for me, my family and my children given my current time, money, energy and other resources. Do I find it easy to follow the "ideal" recipes and other information presented here?

Never!

Do I feel that without at least knowing what the best option is, I have more control over our long-term health and wellness?

Always!

I expect nothing more or less from anyone else.

Thank you for allowing me to stand on my "soap box" regarding sugar! Now, here is my list of "sweet" ingredient options in the order from worst to best.

Worst to Best Countdown of Sweeteners Overview

8. TABLE SUGAR, CANE SUGAR, CANE JUICE, ORGANIC SUGAR CANE, TURBANADO, BROWN SUGAR

Name them whatever you want, the CSID body recognizes them as SUCROSE (TABLE SUGAR).

Even with Sucraid in hand, choosing foods containing minimally processed versions of sugar also contain less chemicals, and less potential to harm. At the time of this edition, it is my understanding that non-gmo cane juice or organic coconut sugar are the least processed forms of sucrose.

7. SPLENDA (SUCRALOSE), NUTRASWEET (ASPARTAME), EQUAL (SACCHARINE)

I avoid using these artificial sweeteners at all costs. The bottom line is they are created for and manufactured for people desiring to continue bad eating habits despite being overweight, having diabetes or worse. Splenda gets my worst of the worst review for their highly deceptive marketing campaign.

Essentially Splenda (or sucralose) is non-corn syrup, sugar based sweetener which is coated in MALTODEXTRIN (starch) to prohibit absorption into the bloodstream. This is no better or healthier than Aspartame, a "sugar substitute", and though research demonstrates small amounts are harmless to adults, the impact on children with existing health problems is unknown. If you feel you must choose a food containing any of the above ingredients, I beg you to consider how necessary the given food is at all?

I provide recipe and food alternatives in this book and on my blog. Consider the benefits of choosing those and reduce the potential harmful effects that artificial sweeteners and sugar substitutes can have on delicate digestive systems. As you will see, there are so many BETTER options if you just look for them.

6. CORN SYRUP OR HIGH FRUCTOSE CORN SYRUP (HFCS)

You would have to be living in a cave to be unaware of all the controversy surrounding corn syrup and high fructose corn syrup. There was a time when I let my guard down and allowed corn syrup and HFCS into Parker's diet. This came in handy when eating out or at social functions when the only beverage available was the lemon-lime soda brand which used corn syrup and no sucrose as a sweetener.

However, I quickly regretted making this compromise as it gave Parker a "taste" for artificial and processed foods. Aside from this, what is the harm? Beyond potentially harming the liver (see footnote on the next page) and leading to other health problems such as diabetes and obesity, most foods containing corn syrup or HFCS are void of any significant nutritional value.

I also read an article describing a more detailed explanation of the differences between corn syrup, HFCS and sugar[4]. Shockingly, this article reveals that some forms of HFCS also contain sucrose!

5. CRYSTALLINE FRUCTOSE

Fructose is a single molecule (monosaccharide) sweeter derived from corn. Though fructose occurs naturally in most fruits, it is my experience that any dried fructose you find in the store comes from corn. Due to its similar taste and consistency to sugar fructose is often one of the first options to use as a sweetener for those with CSID. However, recent reports from Harvard Medical School[5] indicate that high levels of fructose in the diet can contribute to liver problems.

My impression is that this article is pointing toward the high consumption of high fructose corn syrup in processed foods and how the levels of consumption have increased dramatically since the day when our main source of fructose came from fruits. I encourage you to read the article yourself and come to your own conclusion regarding total fructose

---

[4] "The Facts About Corn Syrup". SFChronicle, Sept. 24, 2008.

[5] Skerrett, P.J. *Is Fructose Bad For You?*. Harvard Health Blog. April 26, 2011. Retrieved April 1, 2012 from http://www.health.harvard.edu/blog/is-fructose-bad-for-you-201104262425

intake. A link to this article is available on my blog under the blog post with the same title as this chapter.

Over the past several years I've transitioned from using fructose to sweeten my coffee, tried agave syrup for a time, and after learning of the possible harm of excess fructose, began using Coconut Sugar (see below). I generally only use fructose for baking or cooking if my sweetener of choice (honey) does not compliment to overall flavor or consistency of the recipe or meal.

Please Note: Some people with CSID also lack the enzymes to break down fructose. Consult your dietitian to determine if fructose is the best sugar-substitute for your individual case.

4. STEVIA OR TRUVIA
I've been asked a lot about using Stevia instead of sugar. Honestly, the main thing I don't like about Stevia is that it tastes strange. It's also very expensive to use for baking if used in the quantities needed for the recipes on this blog. However, on occasion and in small quantities (such as to sweeten coffee or tea), I personally use it over artificial sweetener or a sucrose.

Since Stevia is an herb and I have heard from various sources that children should not take in large amounts of herbs (specifically medicinal) I have avoid using it for my children. There just isn't enough long-term use to convince me it is safe. Stevia does not contain sugars of any form. In addition, the ingredients in Truvia are questionable, especially since one is "natural flavors".

One final note to consider if choosing Stevia or Truvia is that this is marketed as a no-calorie sweetener. Since our children require a daily minimum of calories from carbohydrates (a sugar alternative being one of them), this sweetener of choice doesn't add to their caloric needs.

3. AGAVE NECTAR
To the best of my knowledge, agave nectar contains only fructose (up to 90%) and glucose. I have personally used agave nectar to sweeten my coffee and as a last resort to sweeten Parker's chlorophyll or other beverages.

This is one of those products that has recently become a popular sugar substitute. Choose a brand that is known for quality ingredients and processing. I have heard rumors through helpful clerks at local health-food markets that some agave manufacturers may add corn syrup to help stretch their product.

This may turn out to be a great sweetener of choice for those with CSID, but without more research or confirmed reports of successful use, I will leave it up to you to decide. In addition, since it is a form of fructose, you may wish to consider overuse in conjunction with the research about high-fructose corn syrup.

I successfully used a bulk-variety blue agave I purchased from Costco for about two years. I used it mostly in my coffee and in some baking and cooking and cannot recall any digestion problems in using it. I have also used it for traveling when fructose is not available.

If you use it in recipes, I suggest using half the measurement of honey, since it is significantly sweeter.

I prefer agave nectar over crystallized fructose because it's organic, not derived from GMO corn and it's more readily available at grocery stores. However, processing techniques are questionable so I don't consider it as natural an alternative as I once believed.

2. COCONUT SUGAR

I wish I could explain why this form of sucrose doesn't appear to bother those in my family, but I can't. Perhaps it is like certain forms of starch, and simply easier to break down. I've been using it fairly consistently in my coffee for a little over a year now and haven't experienced any issues that I'm aware of.

My kids also prefer the taste over honey in baked treats. Daily intake is very minimal—less than 15 grams and if Parker eats anything containing it, he takes his digestive enzymes just in case.

1. HONEY

Perhaps I am a little partial to honey since it was the only sweetener I ever knew as a child. My mother made us honey sweetened carob cake with whole-wheat flour (which also probably included eggs from our own hens and raw, whole cow's milk) for our birthdays!

Honey is the least processed of all sweeteners and has been used for many thousands of years longer than any of the other sweeteners listed here. Depending on the source, honey contains a very small percentage of sucrose and maltose and is mostly made up of glucose and fructose.

Out of all the healthy foods I grew up with, honey remains one of the only foods our CSID children and I can have without any side effects.

According to CSIDInfo.com, some CSID families use Sucraid with honey. They state that some do not use honey at all, but do not state why. They also list all sweeteners in detail according to CSID tolerance reports and chemical breakdown.

Please note: *Children under the age of 1 year should not eat honey. Please consult your pediatrician regarding the safety of using of honey in baked goods for children under one year.*

PART 2 - SOLUTIONS

"Courage means to keep working a
relationship, to continue seeking solutions
to difficult problems, and to stay focused
during stressful periods."
Denis Waitley

Roanne King

4 - Diagnosing Food Intolerance

Now that you are aware of some of the symptoms to food intolerance, you can begin to take control of digestive health. For parents, I encourage you to become a careful observer of your child. Note any changes in routine or environment along with changes you are making to your child's diet.

Trust Your Instincts and Don't Give Up!
One of the main purposes I have in writing this book is to bring awareness to doctors and parents about the early warning signs of digestive disorders and food intolerance. The priority first and foremost is to equip parents with the confidence they need to know there is something wrong with their child and that they can do something about it.

If a medical diagnosis is necessary or desired by the parent, keeping careful records will provide credibility and hopefully prompt medical professionals to work more diligently towards a diagnosis. As a result, children will begin to get a positive diagnosis earlier on and avoid the many traumatic consequences of living months or years in pain and malnourishment.

I am extremely grateful for the many doctors and specialists that listened to my concerns about my son. Even though it seemed we would never get a definite diagnosis, they frequently respected my 'mother's instinct', and ordered tests upon my insistence. Given the rarity of CSID (even though diagnosis is becoming more and more common), I can now understand how come it was so difficult to determine.

However, had they heeded my concern regarding Parker's digestion from the beginning, a diagnosis could have been made much earlier. As a result, he had to suffer through many months of malnutrition and seizures. If he had not been taking the seizure medication which contained sucrose, and intensified his symptoms, it could have been many more months before he had a diagnosis.

Between the expense and evasiveness of medical tests, some parents may throw up their hands and say "it's not worth it!" My son had numerous tests conducted over the first two years of his life. These tests were highly traumatic and evasive, and almost always induced numerous breath-holding spells and seizures. As his mother, I hated to see him suffer, but I felt I had no other course of action. In addition, many of the tests are expensive and may not be covered by insurance.

For families without insurance, getting a medical diagnosis can cause hardship or seem impossible. Do what you can to receive a firm diagnosis so that you can take the proper and informed action to help your child to the best of your ability. If resources limit your ability to achieve a medical diagnosis, you can still learn to eliminate possible problem foods and environmental factors through careful observation and recording symptoms. My record keeping, insistence, and God's perfect timing ultimately led to the final test of a small bowel biopsy.

I believe both Western Medicine and alternative medicine practices have played a major role in helping my son thrive post-diagnosis. Without the CSID diagnosis, I might still be feeding Parker foods that could harm him and my adult daughter would have no idea which foods to avoid while away at college. Without alternative medicine to guide me in strengthening Parker's digestive system through supplementation and balancing his diet, he may still be struggling with slow growth or malabsorption or worse.

A CSID diagnosis made it easier to know which foods to eliminate and which foods to start with. By adding digestive support supplements and offering Parker a balanced diet despite his food limitations, we experienced many victories despite our many challenges. I won't deny at times it was discouraging to think of all the limitations in his diet, but when I started seeing the positive results, I had the strength to continue down a path to healing (not curing). In the end, I am grateful that I finally have the confidence to know I am truly doing all I can to bring my child to a healthy state. As a result, I am now able to pass on my experience and knowledge in order to benefit other families facing the challenges associated with managing the CSID diet.

Diet Diary, & Symptom Journal

Diagnosing food intolerance is far more difficult than pinpointing a food allergy. Symptoms can come and go and sometimes a change in diet can appear to alleviate the problem for a short time. This is what happened to Parker, when he transitioned from breast milk to formula. His weight gain may have only been water retention and not a healthy sign of growth. It is possible his symptoms seemed to disappear because his body was adjusting to the new form of carbohydrates in the formula. (See Breaking the Vicious Cycle by Elaine Gottschall for more on this theory.)

Keeping track of your child's daily diet over several weeks will help to pinpoint which foods may be causing problems over time. This "accumulation" is a difficult concept to understand or explain. This is why keeping a diet journal is an important step, even if you already have a CSID diagnosis. It will assist you in determining maximum tolerance levels for foods containing sugars and starches. One time a piece of pizza won't seem to cause any problems and the next time, your child is buckled over in pain, vomiting or worse. Over days or weeks, immune system stress may surface in subtle ways such as with a runny nose or increased irritability.

Use a spiral notebook or journal to keep track of everything related to behavior, routine, and food intake for several weeks. I know it is a tedious task and may not be possible to do every day. I assure you, when you do begin to note every detail, certain patterns will emerge. When you notice these patterns bring your notes in to the next doctor's appointment and insist that your child's chart be noted in his or her medical record.

I have copies of Parker's medical records through age three. Over and over again, the doctor wrote "at the insistence of the mother" "because of the mother's great concern" ... this test or that test was ordered. It was my mother's instinct and my tenacity to refuse to settle without an explanation for what my son was going through that eventually led to his diagnosis of CSID.

I would often use one side of my notebook for listing foods, supplements, Sucraid, etc. and the other side to "journal" about Parker's day or week. It was here I would conjecture about my own ideas and thoughts and keep a record of his doctor's comments, tests and results. I kept track of when he woke up, how much sleep he got, if he woke up in the middle of the night, his mood upon waking and anything I thought might be the cause of any less than normal behavior or physical abnormalities. I also noted any variations to recipes or supplements (giving more or less), etc.

Sample Journal Entries

Here is a sample journal entry based on a true incident with my son:

February 23, 2009

Parker has gone four days without chlorophyll. We ran out and I have not had a chance to order more. I have also allowed some compromises to his diet due to time and money constraints. He had a lot of cottage cheese at the restaurant yesterday, and now he has developed a rash around his whole mouth. I don't know if this has to do with anything, but he has come into bed with us every night for the past few days. He has also fallen asleep every afternoon and still had no problem initially going to bed. Usually, if he takes a late afternoon nap, he will not fall asleep with his brothers.

March 3, 2009

I took him in to see his naturopath and testing confirmed he was not doing so well. Though we couldn't pinpoint an exact cause, it was clear the combination of excess meats, restaurant food, and not having his chlorophyll and marshmallow root after eating probably pushed his body over the limit. The rash around his mouth indicated stress in his stomach, and intestines. Upon his doctor's recommendation I purchased a new supply of chlorophyll plus eliminated meats temporarily until his system recovered. She thinks the cottage cheese might be too much for his system right now. I had a hunch, but he just loves it so much! He took the news very well and has been amazingly cooperative. Within two days of implementing diet changes plus supplements, his rash began to clear. He has also slept through the night for the past two days.

Journaling in this instance helped me to discover a hidden warning sign to my son's body being under stress. Now I know it is a possibility that excess sleepiness during the day and restlessness at night might indicate a needed change to his diet. I may never have connected the two possibilities if I wasn't taking notes of every change in behavior. I also realized how important chlorophyll and marshmallow root were to Parker's routine.

Topics to Cover in Journal Entries (Recap)

- mood upon awaking
- doctor appointment details, including height, weight and age
- changes in supplements, medications and why
- number of bowel movements with description of color, smell, and consistency
- number of wet diapers, or urinations
- any foods eaten at restaurants, or from packages (keep labels to record ingredients and to share with your dietitian)
- nap detail (times, how long, differences in normal routine)
- exposure to non-routine cleaning supplies or chemicals (these can cause headaches, irritability, runny nose, cough, etc. and compromise the immune system as well)
- details about developing or continuing rashes
- fever, vomiting or other 'cold' symptoms
- changes in normal mood (i.e., more fussy, tired, hyper, distracted, defiant, etc.)
- questions or thoughts you have about how foods are affecting your child, what to ask the doctor or dietitian, etc.

Diagnosing CSID

There are great efforts being made to improve the ways in which CSID is medically diagnosed. As of the date of publication, I am aware of four methods.

- Two variations of a small bowel biopsy

- Elimination diet (which isn't always accurate as symptoms can also be an indication of fructose intolerance)
- Sucrase Hydrogen Breath Test (limited availability per region and does not indicate starch intolerance levels)
- Sucraid Therapeutic Trial- where a child or adult uses Sucraid (Sacrosidase) with foods containing sucrose. If symptoms improve, some doctors tentatively diagnose CSID while others conduct a biopsy as well.

Please refer to www.csidinfo.com for more information regarding diagnosis of CSID, as well as a more in-depth description of symptoms, sweeteners, sucrose and starch in foods, and lists of doctors familiar with CSID.

NOTE ABOUT SUCRAID ENZYME THERAPY

Sucraid is an enzyme therapy specifically designed to assist those with CSID in digesting SUCROSE ONLY. Sometimes doctors and patients are misled in believing that Sucraid will solve all digestion problems. This is not the case! Sucraid must be prescribed by a doctor -- IF you're fortunate enough to have insurance coverage and access to it.

Since Sucraid only helps in digesting sucrose, and not starches, the second and often missed step is to eliminate starches until sucrose has been gradually and successfully introduced into the diet. Sucraid also only assists in digesting a limited amount of sucrose per meal, up to 25 grams at best.

For more information on Sucraid, dosing and ordering, please see www.sucraid.net

If you are not able to get Sucraid at this time, simply stay with the Group A (See Induction Diet in the next chapter for group definitions) foods that do not require Sucraid. If you are able to determine that your child can tolerate some starch, most of the almond flour recipes should also be safe to use as long as you omit any ingredients marked for use with Sucraid.

5 - The Induction Diet

It is very important to be monitored by a dietitian during the induction diet phase. Your dietitian may add or omit foods based on individual needs. The induction diet is intended to remove all foods from the diet that could be causing digestive issues and to allow the body to recover from the inflammation, irritation and malabsorption resulting from undigested food.

Preparing for the Induction Diet
There are several CSID phenotypes. This is an area where I have not had time to research in addition to the needs of my own family. I suggest that you refer to www.csidinfo.com/InductionDiet.htm for the most recent list of foods for each week.

There are now at least eight known phenotypes, making determining tolerance to starch and sucrose difficult if not impossible. I recommend that you combine the information from the csidinfo site along with your direct observations, diet diary and the recommendation of your pediatrician and dietitian based on enzyme levels.

Understanding Biopsy (Enzyme Level) Results
I feel it is useful and important to note my own children's enzyme levels. In addition, I am including normal levels for digestive enzymes for you to compare with your own child's results. This information will serve as a reference point for your dietitian as you determine which foods and recipes are suitable.

Both of my children started out as Group B and transitioned into Group C sometime around the age of five.

Normal and Abnormal Ranges Are as Follows

Lactase Normal Range: 16.5-32.5; Abnormal: below 16
Sucrase Normal Range: 29-79.8; Abnormal: below 25
Maltase Normal Range: 98-223.6; Abnormal: below 100
Palatinase Normal Range: 4.6-17.6; Abnormal below 5

Results for Parker, age 18 months at the time of testing:
Lactase: 30.4
Sucrase: 6.6
Maltase: 39.0
Palatinase: 0

Results for Elora, age 14 years at the time of testing:
Lactase: 21.1
Sucrase: 2.3
Maltase: 50.4
Palatinase: 2.3

Recall from the introduction that Elora showed symptoms of food intolerance from birth; only breastfed for three months; presented symptoms until age five plus secondary symptoms of soiled pants and bedwetting through age nine; and also experienced a *trauma* at age 14; during which time her symptoms seemed to come back or become more prevalent.

Also, note that her maltase enzymes are higher than Parker's. This supports the theory that those in Group B will be able to tolerate more starch as their digestive system matures[6]. On the contrary, her lactase enzymes are lower. This fact supports the theory that ingesting intolerable foods over a long period of time can stress the lactase enzyme

---

NOTE

Use of the Induction Diet may be needed at various times in your child's life, such as after an infection requiring use of antibiotics or after accidentally ingesting high levels of problem foods that result in extreme symptoms such as diarrhea, vomiting, or weight loss. My children have also experienced faster recovery times by increasing their chlorophyll and digestive supplements after ingesting taboo foods.

---

[6] See www.csidinfo.com for more details.

production process and create a secondary intolerance to lactose, either permanent or temporary[7].

Further Preparation

1. Begin with Group A fruits & vegetables that do not require the use of digestive enzymes. In addition, include unsweetened shredded coconut, unsweetened coconut milk, plain yogurt, cooked eggs, cooked chicken, chicken broth and fish until symptoms subside. An abbreviated list of foods for the first phase of the induction diet begins on the following page.

2. Remove additional dairy products, with the exception of infant formula or breast milk. If you are still breastfeeding, do not add supplemental formula as this interferes with the health of gut flora. Continue to breastfeed as long as possible in order to provide many long term health and digestive benefits[8].

3. It is very important that no additional carbohydrates are allowed. Part of the induction diet process involves starving the harmful bacteria that has been thriving on undigested carbohydrates. This includes artificial sweeteners which can affect pH levels and include maltodextrin. Once this bacterium is gone, "cravings" for harmful carbohydrates should cease.

4. Add digestive-support supplements as listed in chapter 6 and as recommended by a health practitioner such as probiotics, and enzymes. Add a liquid or powder multivitamin that does not contain sugar or starch in any form.

INDUCTION DIET PHASE 1

Foods That Do Not Require Enzymes

---

[7] See *Breaking the Vicious Cycle* by Elaine Gottschall
[8] "Supplementation of the Breastfed Baby: 'Just One Bottle Won't Hurt;--or Will It?" by Marsha Walker, RN, IBCLC

The following meals and food lists do not account for age appropriate foods for infants and toddlers. Consult your health practitioner or dietitian for the proper time to introduce certain foods. This is not an exhaustive list, just a starting place based on the foods I've discovered are easy to digest and contain maximum nutrition.

- Avocados, raw
- Beans, butter, cooked
- Blueberries, frozen or fresh
- Broccoli, steamed
- Cabbage, white, cooked
- Cauliflower, steamed
- Celery, raw
- Coconut; unsweetened shredded, unsweetened milk (
- Cranberries, raw (not dried)
- Cucumber, raw, peeled
- Grapes, white raw
- Kale, steamed
- Lemon, juice
- Lemon, raw
- Lettuce, raw
- Mushrooms, raw
- Spinach, raw
- Tomatoes
- Zucchini (summer squash)
- Plain yogurt
- Eggs
- Poultry
- Fish (3 servings per week needed), salmon, tilapia or canned tuna without soy flakes, broth or starch
- Butter and/or coconut oil for cooking and baking

Keep a diet diary to isolate any problem foods and to keep track of symptoms. Continue using these foods from a balanced approach (1/2 fruits and vegetables, 1/4 animal products, 1/4 yogurt) **until symptom-free for 3 weeks.** For a list of "symptoms" see chapter 1.

Limit fluids during meals to no more than 4 ounces of water with fresh squeezed lemon, agave and liquid chlorophyll. Peppermint tea sweetened with honey, agave, or stevia is also okay. Absolutely no juice of any kind until diarrhea has ceased!

Meal, food and snack items can include:

Breakfast Options
- Scrambled eggs with chopped spinach, mushrooms.
- Plain yogurt with mashed blueberries and fructose/honey.
- Coconut Flour Crepes with mashed berries and yogurt (some find that coconut flour isn't well tolerated at this point).

Lunch Options
- Plain yogurt and frozen blueberry smoothie with added flax oil and powdered vitamins.
- Sliced ripe avocado with albacore tuna (no added starch) and plain yogurt.

Dinner Options
- Cooked butter beans (if canned, make sure only salt added) with chopped tomato
- Chicken breast strips cooked in coconut oil, steamed broccoli
- Salmon burger (no sugar or starch additives) with butter fried zucchini slices and parmesan cheese
- Turkey burger with steamed carrots and butter.

Snacks or Variations
- Use kale or broccoli in scrambled eggs
- Cranberries cooked in water and fructose
- Steamed cabbage with butter
- Hard boiled eggs, chopped or sliced

INDUCTION DIET PHASE 2

Once symptoms are no longer present, fruits containing small amounts of sucrose or requiring Sucraid or digestive enzymes containing invertase can be added. There should be no diarrhea, excess gas, bloating, or rashes present for a full three weeks before beginning this phase.

If Sucraid is not available, do not include the foods in this section unless your health practitioner or dietitian has recommended another supplement containing invertase (enzyme which digests sucrose). Instead, move onto Phase 3 foods, an omit foods which require invertase.

Begin by adding **no more than 5 grams of sucrose per serving, per day with Sucraid or other digestive enzyme containing invertase as recommended by your health practitioner or dietitian**, working up to 5 grams sucrose per meal with Sucraid, then moving to 10 grams sucrose per day, etc.

From this point on, all foods requiring Sucraid or enzymes containing invertase are marked by an *S* for easy reference throughout recipes. The beginning of this phase should only include foods with the lowest levels of sucrose per 100 grams.

Use a food scale for best results. Otherwise, start with very small serving sizes based on your best estimates. This phase will likely involve trial and error, and requires supervision by a dietitian to monitor weight and other factors.

Phase 2 foods include Phase 1 foods plus the addition of:

- Strawberries, raw; Sucrose 1.15
- Raspberries, raw; Sucrose 1.4
- Leaks, raw, Sucrose 1.1
- Apple juice, 100% unsweetened; Sucrose 1. 7
- Onion, raw; Sucrose 2.4
- Apples, raw unpeeled, Sucrose 3.3
- Kiwi; Sucrose 1.7
- Orange, raw; Sucrose 4.1
- Pears, raw; Sucrose 3.67
- Pineapple, raw; Sucrose 6.7
- Carrots, raw; Sucrose 3.02
- Mango, raw; Sucrose 9.7
- Melon, cantaloupe; Sucrose 1.3
- Melon, honeydew; Sucrose 4.9
- Watermelon; Sucrose 3.0

The numbers following each food represent total grams of sucrose per 100 grams.

INDUCTION DIET PHASE 3

By this time, foods known to be tolerated by Group (phenotype) A, using Sucraid as indicated, should be included. As you and your dietitian recommends, begin adding additional dairy foods such as hard cheese, cottage cheese, and sour cream as well as recipes which include almond flour.

At this point, you will be an expert on which foods are tolerated and in what quantities. Remember, CSID symptoms often result from an excess of certain foods over days or weeks. Keep portions small, use digestive enzymes with every meal and snack if you are unsure about the ingredients, and take note of any accumulation of certain foods over several weeks. If exceptions or excess of a particular form of carbohydrate have been ingested, symptoms may resurface. Return to Group A foods or Induction Diet phase 1, until symptoms cease for at least 10 days.

Phase 3 foods include both Phases 1 and 2 foods plus:

- Almonds, raw: 7 grams sucrose; 7 grams starch per 145 gram serving.
- Bananas, *S* Sucrose 6.5 (however green-tipped bananas contain more starch whereas spotted bananas are mostly fructose and sucrose). Begin with 1/3 banana plus enzymes each day working up to a whole banana when 15 grams of sucrose are tolerated. You may need to experiment with varied degrees of ripeness to determine maximum tolerance load per individual.
- Cardamom, ground spice
- Cheese, block such as cheddar or jack (pre-shredded contains potato starch)
- Cheese, soft such as ricotta or mozzarella
- Cottage cheese (without maltodextrin or added starches)

- Cream cheese (if no lactose intolerance, without maltodextrin or added starches)
- Garlic. 1 gram sucrose, 8 grams starch per 28 grams.
- Nutmeg, ground spice
- Pumpkin, raw. 7 grams starch per 245 gram serving.[9]
- Raisins, dried. 27 grams starch per 165 gram serving.
- Sour cream (Daisy brand contains no fillers)
- Squash, buttercup. 18 grams starch per 205 gram serving.
- Walnuts, raw. 3 grams sucrose. 5 grams starch per 117 grams serving
- Flax seed, freshly ground and slowly introduced 1 teaspoon daily added to smoothies, pancakes, crepes or other baked items. 2 grams fiber, no sucrose or starch per 1 tablespoon serving.

It is very important to work with a dietitian during this process. These are only suggestions based on what has helped my family. The final decision of what and when to begin specific foods should be between you and your doctor. Keeping detailed record of diet and additional symptoms is the most accurate way to determine individual tolerance levels.

In summary, however, most of the recipes in this book should be tolerated with the use of a complete digestive enzyme supplement as indicated if the following conditions apply:

1. No other food allergies or intolerance are present, including lactose intolerance.
2. All phases of the induction diet are completed successfully with at least three weeks without stomach upset or other primary symptoms.

---

[9] Starch calculations determined by total carbohydrate less sugars and fiber based on www.nutritiondata.self.com

Even if it appears that certain foods are not tolerated now, you may be able to add it at a later time once symptoms are under control. After my son was virtually symptom-free and gaining weight steadily, I was able to add most of the Group A foods plus almond-flour and dairy products.

As indicated in the title of this book, I have worked diligently to ensure that the foods and recipes mentioned are appropriate for starting to manage a diet void of disaccharides, or excess sucrose and starch. In time, individual tolerance levels may include many more foods, such as starchy vegetables, sweeter fruits, and some grains.

I encourage you to include the insights and recipes provided in this book as much as possible. It is my belief that the CSID diet I present contains some of the healthiest foods on the planet, regardless of digestive limitations.

6 - Digestive Support Supplementation

In today's world, we are all constantly bombarded by free radicals, those nasty little things that love to cause harm to our bodies through promoting disease and debilitating set-backs such as headaches and fatigue. If we don't take measures to assist our bodies in fighting off these mechanisms, disease can ravage our bodies and prevent us from living healthy, productive lives. For a growing child who has already faced many health challenges, strengthening and supporting his or her digestive system is a key factor to bringing balance to all major body systems.

Through understanding digestive enzyme deficiencies and experiencing the positive changes associated with including digestive-support supplementation, my family has many less woes and can recover more quickly if we break the rules and eat a taboo food.

I came into the knowledge of many of these supplements from either my son's dietitian or his naturopathic doctor. This is only a partial list of the dozens of digestive-support and body-system- strengthening products available. My family has personally experienced the benefits of using the ones listed in this book, and I have seen marked improvement in my son since implementing these into his already sugar-and-starch- free diet.

After just one year of diligently administering the below supplements, Parker gained 5 pounds and grew 5 inches! It was the most he had ever grown at one interval, and the first time he began to show a promising upward slant to his own growth curve. His constant runny nose and reoccurring cough was gone. In addition, his overall countenance improved. He became a happy, outgoing, talkative child and though he is still a year behind in size from other eight-year-olds, his size does not hold him back one bit.

There is no way of knowing which combination of these supplements has improved Parker's health the most. I am sure many of them compliment and assist each other. Each child's needs and the level of stress in their digestive system will vary. We have not always had the financial means to keep our shelves stocked, and once Parker was doing well for period of time, many of these supplements needed.

rient and Digestion Support

Shaklee vitamins, supplements, and cleaning p. over 15 years. Their quality is superb and I highly recommend you find a local distributor or take advantage of their wholesale membership offers. Anything not offered through Shaklee, I order through Nature's Sunshine, another long-lived company that also specializes in digestive health.

Upon careful consideration of ingredients and additives, you have a gamut of alternatives to enzymes and digestive support supplements available through online retailers. A few retailers and brands I've learned to trust include:

www.shaklee.com
www.naturessunshine.com
www.worldnutrition.com
www.gardenoflife.com
www.kirkmanlabs.com
www.klaire.com
www.energeticnutrition.com

- A liquid, powdered or chewable **multivitamin** without added sugar such as Shaklee Infant Powder or Incredivites, is essential.
- **Omega-3** supplement such as added flax-oil to yogurt or smoothies.
- **Probiotics** that do not include added sucrose (sugar), sucralose or starch. Recognition of the benefits of probiotics, especially for those with digestive disorders is becoming more accepted and recommended in mainstream medicine. Parker uses Nature's Sunshine "Sunshine Heroes Probiotic Power" chewable tablets.

For younger children, mashing supplements or blending works if they will not or cannot swallow tablets or capsules.

Below I have listed the supplements I regularly used with cooking and baking for Parker through age five.

DIGESTIVE SUPPORT SUPPLEMENTS

Liquid Chlorophyll

According to Nature's Sunshine, chlorophyll is a "ais tract detoxifier", "supports intestinal health", and "supports circulatory health".

There was a point in his early CSID days that the only liquid Parker had was his cup of chlorophyll mixed with distilled water, honey and lemon. I believe having this supplement consistently allowed his digestive system to recover from months of malabsorption as well as to get over bouts of diarrhea within days or even hours.

Compared to the three weeks it can takes some children with CSID to recover from accidentally ingestion of too many sugars or starches, this is definitely a supplement I recommend! My son knows it helps him and will ask for his chlorophyll when his tummy is bothering him.

Another purpose for using liquid chlorophyll with the CSID diet is to strengthen the immune system and bring pH balance to the body. Take 1-2 teaspoons in 6 ounces distilled or purified water with half a squeezed lemon. Sweeten with fructose, stevia or honey. Sip on 2-4 cups in any given day. Find it at www.naturessunshine.com.

See the recipe for Chlorophyll Cocktail in PART 3.

Papaya Mint or Chewable Super Papaya Enzyme Plus

These chewable tablets contain papaya enzymes, mint, and depending on the brand also contain chlorophyll and other enzymes. The enzymes primarily break down proteins, stimulate digestive juices, and may assist in breaking down lactose. Parker uses Nature's Sunshine "Sunshine Heroes Chewable Papaya Enzymes." Note that these enzymes contain sorbitol and fructose.

Kirkman Carbdigest™ With Isogest® Capsules

Aids in the digestion of carbohydrates, specifically isomaltose.

Order from Kirkmanlabs.com

Nature's Sunshine Food Enzyme Capsules

Used by me and my adult daughter, these provide a blend of enzymes to digest proteins, carbohydrates (up to 25 grams of starch) and fats. Enter "Food Enzymes" in search box online.

Klaire Labs Vital-Zymes™ Chewable
Chewable enzymes containing carbohydrate-specific enzymes: amylase, alpha-amylase, glucoamylase with isomaltase side chain activity; sugar-specific enzymes: lactase, sucrose (invertase), maltase, pullulnase (debranching enzyme with isomaltase side chain activity), and vegetable/plant fiber specific enzymes (cellulose, and hemicellulase/pectinase/phytase complex). Available through various retailers on Amazon.

Distilled Water
Drinking distilled water in small amounts (no more than 4oz every half-hour) throughout the day is important in assisting the vital organs to filter out toxins, bacteria, and harmful salts. It may also help to bring the body to its ideal alkaline state. Most grocery stores sell distilled water in gallon-sized bottles.

Use distilled water as a base for use with liquid chlorophyll and lemon. You may notice better results by taking fluids in small amounts at regular intervals. This ensures hydration and reduces stress to the liver and kidneys that may occur from excess fluid intake.

As an added step, you may wish to drain canned vegetables and butter beans, soak them in distilled water, and then rinse to remove sodium and any residuals from the water they are canned in.

Magnesium
In the beginning, magnesium supplementation was a vital component to Parker's supplement plan. Often one of the first nutrients depleted when the body is under stress, magnesium helps prevent constipation, eases muscle strain (which can cause headaches), increases energy and assists in bringing the body into an alkaline state.

There are several brands of magnesium available through health food stores and distributors in liquid, capsule, or tablet form. If swallowing capsules is difficult, you can mix powder from capsules or liquid versions into foods such as yogurt or smoothies.

Read labels carefully and avoid supplements containing fillers or ingredients which may include sucrose or starch. Consult your doctor or dietitian regarding proper dosage. Take with food.

Marshmallow Root (Althaea Officinalis)
There are properties in the marshmallow root that may assist the body in eliminating harmful substances quickly. It can strengthen mucus membranes and the respiratory system and eases gastrointestinal irritation. Upon approval of your doctor/dietitian, begin with 1 or 2 capsules after a meal. If tolerable, dissolve capsules in warm water and serve with each meal.

This product has also done wonders for other family members (including myself) after eating meals with an excess of starches or sugars. Available through Nature's Sunshine and other natural food retailers.

There are dozens if not hundreds of digestive-support types of supplements available on the market. I have listed the above supplements and nutrients based on my own personal experience, recommendations by my son's naturopathic doctor and dietitian, and because of the marked improvement in his health upon regularly including them in his already sugar-free, low-starch diet.

L-Glutamine Powder (New)
Traditionally used as a supplement for recovery after intense exercise, it can also be used to help the intestine recover after digestive distress. I added this product to Parker's supplements while working to help him combat eczema. We added ½ teaspoon of the powder to diluted 100% grape juice 1-2 times per day. I believe the inclusion of L-Glutamine powder was one factor in Parker overcoming his food allergies in 2015.

SYSTEMIC ENZYMES SUPPORT (New)
I've recently learned about the importance of systemic enzyme support for overall health. Systemic enzymes work throughout the body to support all systems, eliminate waste,

and reduce scar tissue among their thousands of other processes.

When a body is under addition stress (such as a digestive enzyme deficiency), systemic enzymes are also depleted. This lack of systemic support may also lead to the variety of symptoms associated with malabsorption, such as fatigue, headaches, mood issues and more. Ideally, systemic enzymes should only be taken with water at least an hour between meals. This may present an issue for small children, but older children and adults can still benefit. The brand of Systemic Enzymes that my family has used with success is World Nutrition's Vitalzym Extra Strength (not to be confuses with Klaire Labs) available at EnergeticNutrition.com. I highly recommend discussing the addition of systemic enzymes with your health practitioner or dietitian.

7 - Breastfeeding and First Foods

Breastfeeding and Digestive Health[10]
To date, there is no documented research indicating that children with CSID present any symptoms prior to beginning solid foods. However, my son Parker DID show signs of failure to thrive, suffered from seizures and presented other symptoms related to CSID long before he had anything but breast milk.

According to some studies on breast milk, the oligosaccharides found in human breast milk can reduce or prevent diarrhea[11]. This information got me to thinking how my son, Parker, never had full-blown diarrhea, though his BMs were always oily, very smelly, and bulky compared to my other breastfed children. As many of you mothers out there know, breastfed infants rarely produce smelly BMs. Usually the "stink starts" when other food is introduced!

Though CSID cannot be prevented by breastfeeding, studies suggest that it can definitely protect children from developing other digestive diseases or infections due to an imbalanced gut. There is already proof that breastfeeding can have a "protective effect" on children susceptible to Celiac Disease[12].

Looking back to just before Parker was diagnosed with CSID, I recall the week before seeing his GI he was very sick and lethargic. He was having several BMs, several in an hour at times, but nothing that appeared to be diarrhea. After receiving his diagnosis, I discovered that many children with CSID are hospitalized due to dehydration. Though Parker

---

[10] Rehmeyer, Julie J. "Milk Therapy: Breast Milk Compounds Could Be a Tonic for Adult Ills." *Science News.* 170.24. December 9, 2006. p. 376.Retrieved from Infotrac Custome 750 Journals on February 1, 2012.

Walker, Marsha, RN, IBCLC. "Supplementation of the Breastfed Baby: Just One Bottle Won't Hurt, or Will It?" N.D.

[11] Miller, Janette Brand. McVeagh, Patricia. "Human Milk Oligosaccharides: 130 Reasons to Breastfeed." *British Journal of Nutrition,* 1999. pp. 333-335.

[12] Ayers, Art. Breastfeeding Decreases Celiac and Diabetes: Weaning After First Foods Protects Against Autoimmune Diseases. December 26, 2008.

was hospitalized several times, the reason was always due to his seizures, not dehydration by malabsorption.

I breastfed Parker until he was about 14 months old, adding only some solid food at nine months (most of which I removed from his diet since nearly everything seemed to exacerbate or increase his symptoms). I fully credit the benefits of breast milk as the sole reason he was never hospitalized for dehydration. However, breastfeeding may also have been the reason for his delayed diagnosis given it may have prevented the severe diarrhea that would have demanded the doctor's attention!

Although this theory surrounding my own child's connection between CSID symptoms and breastfeeding is not conclusive, my hope is that you will let me know if you experienced a similar situation. If we can band together and share our stories related to breastfeeding (or not) and try to find a connection, we may help that child and mother facing undiagnosed digestive issues.

First Foods for Infants and Toddlers

PLEASE NOTE THIS LIST DOES NOT ACCOUNT FOR ADDITIONAL FOOD INTOLERANCE (SUCH AS LACTOSE) OR ALLERGIES

*For infants, steam, mash or puree with breast milk, formula, plain yogurt, almond milk or coconut milk at your pediatrician's recommendation.

S= Sucraid recommended or required, consult dietitian

Starting with vegetables and non-sweet foods will help in developing a variable palate. Eliminating processed sweets and offering naturally sweet food (such as berries) as an occasional treat is ideal. This will help your child appreciate the treat and demonstrate how sweet foods in moderation will not cause harm.

I highly discourage using commercially prepared baby foods on a regular basis for several reasons.

1. The nutritional content is almost always compromised as foods must be heated at high levels during the packaging process. This heating process removes many vital nutrients.

2. There is no guarantee that added fillers, pesticides or other harmful ingredients (such as sugar) are not present. Food manufacturers are not required to list trace amounts of ingredients or chemicals.

3. Using convenience foods sets up a lifelong habit of consuming "fast food" that will inevitably compromise a healthy, high-quality diet.

4. Save these foods for emergencies or for traveling when absolutely necessary, and always choose single ingredient, organic foods to ensure the highest quality possible.

If you see a traditional "baby food" not listed, such as peas or corn, it is because it contains excess starch. Grains are not listed here due to their high starch content, and the belief of some healthcare professionals that grains can strain developing digestive systems and other organs if offered before the age of two.

However, as you will see, there are still many healthier, easy to prepare foods to choose from! I have noted the approximate age where introducing this food is appropriate as a basic guideline. Consult your child's dietitian to confirm age-appropriate foods.

Exclusive Breastfeeding while Mom eats CSID-friendly foods Until 9 months if Possible

(S) indicates Sucraid is needed.

All vegetables are cooked, mashed and/or cut into bite-sized pieces unless otherwise noted.

9-24 months, BM + Food	6 mos	7 mos	8 mos	9 mos	10 mos	11 mos	1 year	18 mos
							honey may be added to diet	
Vegetables	avocado	carrots (S), green beans, spaghetti squash, zucchini, yellow summer	broccoli	cauliflower, spinach, kale, onions (S), butter beans, mushrooms			bell peppers	cabbage, cucumber (peeled)
Fruits	ripe banana (S) *symptom-free, beginning with 1/3 banana per day*		red or white grapes, cut very small or mashed	blueberries, cherries, strawberries (S)-maybe, pineapple (S), diluted luke warm apple cider (cloudy, fresh pressed)			tomato, lemons or limes, Diluted 100% grape, pomegranate or cranberry juice	
Fruits to serve sparingly, and in very small portions			apple(S), watermelon(S), cantaloupe(S)	pears(S), peaches(S)				

Exclusive Breastfeeding while Mom eats CSID-friendly foods Until 9 months if Possible

(S) indicates Sucraid is needed.

All vegetables are cooked, mashed and/or cut into bite-sized pieces unless otherwise noted.

	6 mos	7 mos	8 mos	9 mos	10 mos	11 mos	1 year	18 mos
Dairy		cottage cheese, ricotta cheese	plain yogurt, hard cheese					
Nuts			blanched almond flour*	coconut milk, almond milk	thinned almond butter		coconut flour, shredded coconut	
Meat, Fish, Poultry		eggs, cooked yolk only	cooked chicken or turkey, beef	whole eggs	salmon, tilapia, tuna, trout	pork		

*Almond flour contains protein, fiber, calcium, magnesium, vitamin E, folate, iron, phosphorus, potassium, biotin, and many more valuable nutrients. It contains very little to no starch in comparison to peanuts and is much easier to digest overall.

8 - Carbohydrate Essentials

The CSID diet is not simply "sugar-free" or "low-carb". These catch phrases used by food manufacturers are deceptive at best and mislead many into assuming foods labeled this way are somehow healthier. Upon hearing that our CSID diet requires the elimination of sugars and starches, one of the first responses I hear is, "So it's like Celiac or the Atkins diet?"

My answer to this is always "yes and no." Yes, the CSID diet is gluten-free since all foods containing gluten also contain starch. Yes, the Atkins diet comes close, but still allows many foods that can cause problems in addition to it being a 'diet' focused on low calorie and low carb living. Calories and carbs are actually an essential part of thriving for those with CSID.

This is the quandary. With only a handful of carbohydrate options, what can our kids eat? Children suffering from malabsorption need carbohydrates to grow.

For children who have failed to grow properly due to digestive problems, carbohydrates are actually a very important part of their nutritional needs. However, the challenge is in providing children with CSID, or disaccharide deficiency, the 45-65% of total calories that should come from carbohydrates.[13]

Low-starch foods that contain high amounts of carbohydrates are difficult to find. The majority of carbohydrates must come from dairy products (if lactose intolerance is not an issue), non-starchy vegetables and fruit containing mostly fructose or glucose. Additional sources of needed carbohydrates must also come from honey, fructose or glucose supplements. Without including these monosaccharides, children may not receive enough carbohydrates to maintain energy or gain weight at a steady rate.

---

[13] www.livestrong.com

The Importance of Digestive Enzyme Supplementation

With the use of digestive enzymes, additional and necessary carbohydrates can be consumed. Talk with your healthcare professional about the digestive enzymes that can work best for your situation. In addition to the prescription enzyme for help with sucrose digestion, Sucraid, there are several other forms of supplements available at health food retailers.

Some of the additional high-carbohydrate foods that can be consumed with enzymes include peaches, pears, bananas, cantaloupe, watermelon, pineapple and high-calorie sauces such as dressings, pasta sauce, and barbeque sauce.

Non-Starchy, High-Carb Vegetables

Non-starchy vegetables that contain higher levels of carbohydrates include mushrooms, kale, cucumber, zucchini, carrots, broccoli, green beans, cauliflower and tomato juice. As you will see, these are the primary foods I use in my recipes.

In addition, avocado, flax oil and coconut oil contain essential fats and can be added to smoothies, baked good or used in cooking.

Starch Tolerance Testing

So how do you know if starches are tolerated starches at all? The small biopsy enzyme test results provided by the GI will be an indicator as to whether any starch will be tolerated. Once there are no symptoms and low weight is not a concern, then the following "starch tolerance test" can be conducted under the supervision of a dietitian.

1. Each individual must go 3 weeks without any starches at all. Even trace amounts can skew the results. Stick with Group A foods—primarily berries, non-starchy vegetables, meat, poultry, fish, eggs, and dairy. No almonds or peanuts allowed.

2. The child must not be underweight, or have had any diarrhea or vomiting for 3 weeks as well,

3. You will need a box of saltine crackers and a notebook.

DAY 1 Note child's weight and the date. Start with 1 saltine cracker in the morning and note the time. Aside from a few sips of water, do not allow child to drink excess fluids when they eat the cracker.

Each square cracker contains approximately 2 grams of starch. Note any symptoms such as bloating, gas, complaints of stomach pain along with the time they occurred. If none, write this down as well and continue with DAY 2 below.

If symptoms do occur, be sure to write down additional liquids and food the child had throughout the day.

Repeat Day 1 again, adjusting other foods and liquids to determine if symptoms were due to a food-combination issue or a starch-tolerance issue. Do not continue to Day 2 if after several tries, a single cracker creates digestive distress. Starch is not appropriate at this time. If no symptoms occur, move to DAY 2.

DAY 2 Repeat Day 1 and add another single cracker at lunch time. Again, if symptoms present themselves, notate additional food and liquids and try 1 cracker in the morning and at lunch time again. If no symptoms occur, move on to DAY 3.

DAY 3 Add a third single saltine cracker to dinner. Note symptoms if any. If none, move to DAY 4.

DAY 4 Beginning on this day, you will increase crackers to 2 per serving, 3 times per day. If no symptoms present themselves, you will continue to increase the number of crackers per meal, per day until symptoms occur. Once symptoms present, the total number of crackers tolerated on the previous day is the total starch tolerance level.

EXAMPLES TEST RESULTS:

- Day 4 (2 crackers per meal, 3 times per day) symptom free = Total Starch Tolerance Level of 4 grams per meal.
- Day 5 (3 crackers per meal, 3 times per day) symptom free = Total Starch Tolerance Level of 6 grams per meal.
- Day 6 (4 crackers per meal, 3 times per day) symptom free = Total Starch Tolerance Level of 8 grams per meal.

- Day 7 (5 crackers per meal, 3 times per day) symptom free = Total Starch Tolerance Level of 10 grams per meal.

This may seem daunting, but it is the best method to determine exactly how much starch is tolerated.

You may add non-starchy toppings that don't require enzyme supplementation to add flavor if needed. Toppings may include cream cheese, pure fruit raspberry jam, plain yogurt with sliced blueberries, avocado slices with sea salt, peeled cucumbers with tuna (if canned, make sure there is no broth or soy flakes added).

Starchy foods that are still easy on digestion include sweet potatoes (orange have higher sucrose content, white have more starch), butternut squash, pumpkin, green peas, and white potatoes (peeled). Consult a dietitian after the starch tolerance test is complete to see if you can add these foods as additional carbohydrate sources.

Estimating Sucrose and Starches Using Nutrition Facts Labels

Nutrition Facts
Serving Size 1/8 of recipe 102g (101 g)

Amount Per Serving	
Calories 227	Calories from Fat 171

	% Daily Value*
Total Fat 20g	30%
Saturated Fat 9g	45%
Trans Fat	
Cholesterol 135mg	45%
Sodium 131mg	5%
Total Carbohydrate 5g	2%
Dietary Fiber 2g	7%
Sugars 1g	
Protein 10g	

Vitamin A	56%	• Vitamin C	33%
Calcium	17%	• Iron	8%

*Percent Daily Values are based on a 2,000 calorie diet. Your daily values may be higher or lower depending on your calorie needs:

		Calories	2,000	2,500
Total Fat	Less than		65g	80g
Sat Fat	Less than		20g	25g
Cholesterol	Less than		300mg	300mg
Sodium	Less than		2,400mg	2,400mg
Total Carbohydrate			300g	375g
Fiber			25g	30g

Calories per gram:
Fat 9   •   Carbohydrate 4   •   Protein 4

©www.NutritionData.com

Nutrition Facts Label for "Breakfast Quiche"

I don't know about you, but I find Nutrition Facts labels confusing when it comes to determining the total starch and sugar content in a packaged food. They isolate the carbohydrates by sugars and fiber. This does not help us much as sugar can stand for sucrose, fructose, glucose, lactose or other forms of sugar. There is a way, however, to use the Nutrition Facts Label in conjunction with the ingredients to estimate how much sucrose and starch a serving of food contains.

First of all, choose foods with very few ingredients whenever possible. The more ingredients the food has, the more daunting this task will become. Consider it a junk-food-proof motivation to stick with mostly pure, unprocessed foods whenever possible!

Next, you will need to memorize all the different names for sugar; primarily anything ending in "-ose", with the exception of fructose and glucose. Unless there is another dietary issue, these monosaccharides (single molecule sugars) can be tolerated by those with CSID. Also, avoid anything containing the words syrup, such as rice syrup and corn syrup. Palm kernel nectar is also over 90% sucrose. Other names for sugar include cane sugar, cane juice, turbinado sugar, brown sugar, and molasses. Please see chapter 3,"Choosing the Best Sugar Substitute" for an overview of all sweeteners.

Generally, the order of the ingredients indicates the percentage of the ingredient used to make the overall product. If sugar is the first word, you should avoid it all together unless total sugars per serving is less than 5 grams.

Please note that experimenting and estimating starch and sugar content in packaged foods should not be attempted during episodes of major symptoms. Ideally, the child or adult should have successfully completed 3 weeks of the Induction Diet without symptoms before adding foods which may contain starch or sugar.

Performing the following steps and calculations will help you to determine if a food is tolerable, as well as how much sugar or starch a serving contains.

1. TOTAL Carbohydrates per serving should be no more than 35 grams. Servings containing carbohydrates higher than this probably contain too much starch for the CSID diet. If starch tolerance levels have not been determined, this number should be far lower. If Sucraid is not available and if any of the ingredients include a form of sugar, this food should be avoided for the time being.

2. Look at the breakdown of sugars and fiber below the carbohydrates. Comparing the ingredients again, search for sources of fiber if the food contains fiber in any amount. Fiber sources which may irritate those with CSID or other digestive problems include wheat, bran, corn, rice, quinoa, potatoes, farina, wheat germ, and others. Only choose foods containing fiber sources from fruits, vegetables, legumes (if they are sprouted) and nuts. If the source of fiber is "safe" (not from a grain), you can then subtract the total fiber from

the total carbohydrates. Using the label above as an example, we now have 3 grams of carbohydrates left to account for.

3. To determine starch content, subtract the total sugars from the remaining carbohydrates. This means a serving of the Breakfast Quiche labeled above has a total of 2 grams of starch per serving. This is an acceptable amount of starch since it most likely comes from the almond flour and possibly the mushrooms.

4. If you want to find out the total sucrose content, you will have to estimate depending on the ingredients. For example, you are looking at a carton of ice cream you can assume that the majority of the total "sugars" is probably from lactose or the milk sugar. Overall, the total sugars per serving taken with Sucraid should not exceed 25 grams.

In Summary:

- No grains or sucrose.
- TOTAL CARBOHYDRATES less than 35grams per serving
- Carbohydrates - fiber = sugar and starch
- Carbohydrates - fiber & sugar = starch
- Remember dairy products containing lactose are counted in the total sugars.
- Group A (or limited maltose enzymes) should not have any starches from grains. Almond flour and fiber from non-sugary fruits or non-starchy vegetables are okay.
- Group C, symptom-free may be able to tolerate up to 35 grams of starch per serving. See "Starch Tolerance Test" to help determine individual tolerance levels.
- Use Food Enzymes or Kirkman Isogest with foods containing more than 5 grams of starch per serving.
- Use Sucraid 1-2ml with foods containing more than 5 grams of sucrose per serving.

Additionally, supplement with Sunshine Heroes Enzymes and Sunshine Heroes Probiotics for maximum digestion support.

PART 3 - RECIPES

"This is fantabulous, Mom! Wonderific!"
Parker, age 5

Roanne King

9 - Getting Started

"Mom, do you like cooking?" My daughter Tayler asked one afternoon as I began pulling out ingredients for a new recipe back in 2008.

"Not really. It's frustrating to spend time and energy cooking something everyone just complains about."

Less than two weeks later Elora's test results came back. She also had CSID in addition to her five-year-old brother!

I took a deep breath, pushing back tears as my mind swarmed with the many struggles I would surely face. Then I had to laugh, recalling Tayler's question. Whether or not I liked cooking, my family needed to learn how to eat differently. I needed to learn to cook the foods that were best for all of us. Elora would be going off to college before I could blink. Besides, all of our kids could potentially have children with CSID one day. Creating good cooking and eating habits would be essential to their future health and the future health of my grandchildren.

No, I don't like cooking or baking. With the exception of doing so with my sisters and mother during the holidays, cooking does not bring me much joy. However, when my little Parker comes up to me and reaches up to wrap his tiny arms around my waist after finishing off a whole plate filled with my latest sugar-less, starch-less meal, I know every bit of my efforts have been worth it!

Here are some things I have found helpful while adjusting to cooking the CSID way. Hopefully these tips will give you needed motivation or help you get through one more day of experimental cooking. Maybe you will also reap a harvest of smiles around the table and requests for a second helping.

1. **Take a deep breath and focus on what you can do today**. With five children, a self-employed husband and my over-achieving personality, I have had to face the very real fact that I cannot do it all. Sometimes I have more money than time. Other days I have more time than money. I don't always plan ahead and often I make compromises as a result.

However, I take comfort in believing each day is a chance for a new beginning.

2. *Make small goals and plan when you can*. As you begin cooking CSID-friendly foods, decide which meals and recipes are most important. If major symptoms are present, take it one day at a time. Replace one meal at a time. Begin with ingredient substitutes (see below), then move onto entire meals. Remove "problem" foods from your child's reach or from your house completely.

3. *Get the whole family involved*. Talk to your spouse, grandparents, and child's siblings about how important diet changes are. Find recipes that closely resemble what your family normally eats. Perhaps you can try desserts first. Recruit older children to help you make a salad, push the button on the blender when making smoothies, or scoop the muffin batter into the muffin tins. Share recipes with extended family or bring enough to share at the next family gathering.

4. *Batch bake to save both time and money*. Some ingredients, such as almond flour, can be very expensive if purchased in small quantities. Now that I have my list of "best recipes" (those I know my kids will eat and that are great for on the go) I know that ordering 5 or even 10 pounds of almond flour will ensure I have plenty on hand to batch bake. Other ingredients that are best to buy in bulk include eggs, butter, honey, fructose and unsweetened coconut. Usually I set aside one morning during the week to batch-bake several recipes at once.

The amount you bake will depend on how much storage space you have in your refrigerator or freezer. The recipes I typically batch bake are coconut macaroons, almond flour muffins or cookies, coconut flour crepes, Knox-blox and lima bean soup. I use them for a quick breakfast, school lunches, after-school snacks or as dessert leverage (yes, bribery!) when experimenting with a new dinner recipe.

5. *Recipe tricks and tips*. Every time I use a recipe, I discover something new. Sometimes I do not have all the

ingredients I need. Other times I realize my dir
tweaking. Some recent examples include:

- Do not use paper cups for muffin or macar
  Almond flour sticks worse than any other flcus; ᴛᴴᴇ ʟast
  few times I have made muffins, I have generously greased
  muffin tins with butter or coconut oil, and left out the
  muffin cups. A silicone or rubber spatula works great to
  remove the muffins as well. I've also found that almond
  flour doesn't stick to parchment paper baking cups. Cool
  for just a few minutes, and then remove muffins to finish
  cooling on a rack.
- For coconut flour or breakfast crepes, make sure the pan
  is hot, butter is melted and that you use just enough
  batter to cover the pan. Make sure the crepe cooks to the
  point of browning, and flip by lifting up just the edge of
  the crepe. Don't try to get the spatula under the entire
  crepe (as you would with a pancake) or the crepe can
  break.
- Cook extra chicken, turkey breast or vegetables. Cube,
  crumble and store for the next day's meals. Cubed
  chicken can be added to salads for lunch. Cooked ground
  turkey and chopped veggies such as broccoli can be
  added to scrambled eggs for breakfast.

6. *Ingredient Substitutes.* Do you ever come across a recipe
in a magazine that looks great, but you're not sure how to
substitute ingredients to make the recipe acceptable for the
CSID diet? Most of my recipes were inspired by traditional
recipes. Some of these exchanges are basic, while others may
not be so obvious.
- Use sea salt instead of regular salt. Even though salt of
  any kind can be digested, the benefits of sea salt are
  becoming so main-stream that many packaged foods now
  boast it as their salt of choice. After exclusively using sea
  salt for the past five or more years, I can now tell a huge
  difference in taste. Sea salt adds an authentic flavor and
  is void of the chemical side effects processed salt can
  create.
- Exchange equal amounts of crystalline fructose for sugar.

Replace other beans, pasta or rice with white cooked lima beans. I usually purchase several cans of lima beans called "butter beans". Be careful to read ingredient lists so that you know no sugar or starches are added. To remove added salt, drain beans and place in a small bowl with enough distilled water to cover beans. Soak for 15 minutes, and rinse in a colander. Then add sea salt to taste after warming. These beans also make a great thickening substitute for cream sauces or soups that normally call for white flour or cornstarch. Simply blend until smooth.

- Almond flour for white flour. Since almond flour has a very different composition than white flour, a direct exchange for a traditional recipe will not work. Generally, almond flour bakes like quick bread. The best alternative I have found is to take one of my almond flour recipes, such as the banana-nut muffins and swap out the "flavor" ingredients. Exchange mashed banana and walnuts for shredded carrots (carrot cake), shredded apples (apple muffins), shredded zucchini, blueberries or strawberries, or grated cheese for a variety of flavors. Almond flour mixed with melted butter is also a great crust substitute for either pizzas or pies.
- Spaghetti squash or cauliflower as a starch substitute. Spaghetti squash can be used for pasta, as a dessert with honey and butter, added to muffins, soups and more. I use cauliflower as a crust substitute (see Hawaiian Pizza), fake mashed potatoes, instead of pasta, flaked with butter instead of rice and more.

Prepare yourself to begin to look differently at the what, why and how your family eats. Having some basic tools in the kitchen can save you time as you transition.

Basic Tools

- Electric Mixer
- Blender and/or Food Processor
- Lemon Juicer
- Glass storage containers
- Glass or Stone Bread loaf pan

- Muffin tins
- Crockpot
- Food dehydrator
- Toaster Oven for baking small batches and reheating food without destroying nutrients.
- Yogurt maker if you suspect lactose intolerance
- Freezer and refrigerator space dedicated to storing prepared foods.

Serving Sizes

Serving sizes are not in accordance with official serving portions according to the USDA. Reference to the amount of servings in these recipes is an estimate based on portions typically used by my family. This is only a rough indicator as to how many servings you may get from a particular recipe and may vary depending on age and preference. Your dietitian will be able to determine proper portions.

You may need to divide measurements for some ingredients, but this chart contains conversions for the temperatures and ingredients in the amounts used for most recipes.

FROM FAHRENHEIT TO CELSIUS*				GENERAL CONVERSION				
	°F	°C		Cup	Fluid Ounce	TBSP	TSP	Milliter
	300	150		1	8	16	48	237
	325	170		3/4	6	12	36	177
	350	180		2/3	5	11	32	158
	375	190		1/2	4	8	32	158
	400	200		1/3	3	5	16	79
	425	220		1/4	2	4	12	59
	450	230		1/8	1	2	6	30

Ounces	Grams
2	50
4	100
6	170
8	230
10	280
12	340
16	450

CUPS TO GRAMS	
Cups	Grams
Almond Flour	
1	100
Berries	
1/2	75
Yogurt	
1	226

OUNCES TO GRAMS	
Ounces	Grams
Mushrooms	
2	50
Cheese	
4	120

CUPS TO MILLILITERS	
Cups	Milliliters
Honey	
1/2	150
Water, Juice or Milk	
1	250
1/2	140

elevation may also effect cooking times

10 - Shopping Lists and Staple Ingredients

There are specific ingredients and product manufacturers I have grown to trust over the years. Read through this list carefully and refer to it often. Make it a habit to ALWAYS check labels, even when using a trusted brand, as I can't guarantee that a particular manufacturer has not changed its ingredients since the date of publication of this book.

There are a few parameters to master when you first start shopping for CSID-friendly foods and ingredients. First and foremost—label reading! Luckily, most of these shopping lists include only single ingredient, fresh foods. For others, becoming aware of which ingredients may present a problem is grueling but worth the effort in the end!

In general, I never trust front label claims such as "all natural" or "sugar-free", as I quickly learned most still include sugar substitutes that can cause secondary symptoms. These include soy products and any form of sugar, including evaporated cane juice.

KEY INGREDIENTS TO AVOID:

Starchy ingredients or association with starchy foods including rice, corn, potato, oats, tapioca, garbanzo bean, peanut, wheat, modified food starch, maltodextrin, soy or soy flakes, high fructose corn syrup, corn syrup, broth or anything labeled "natural flavors". Remember, "low-carb" or "gluten-free" may indicate high starch or sugar content.

Sucrose or artificial sugars including sugar, brown sugar, molasses, cane sugar, cane juice, evaporated can juice, palm sugar or syrup, sucralose (Splenda), aspartame, corn syrup, high fructose corn syrup.

Fiber-Based Irritants include bran, wheat germ, psyllium, quinoa, farina, and small seeds such as whole flax seed, sesame seeds, pumpernickel, poppy seeds, etc. While the bowel is irritated, seeds and grain-based-fiber can get caught in the inflamed tissue and increase irritation and gas.

If you are not sure about an ingredient, it is safer to pass on the particular food. I also learned from several sources that manufacturers are not required to disclose every single ingredient. If I have listed a particular brand name, it is due to the purity of the product, my success in using it, or a specific recommendation from either the SCD diet or the CSID approved foods list.

I have found some of these ingredients very difficult to avoid in certain foods, such as the inclusion of maltodextrin or food starch in most brands of cottage cheese, sour cream and even yogurt. However, there are brands out there that do not add fillers. Keep searching until you find one or purchase a yogurt maker of your own. Even when you do, continue to check labels regularly as manufacturers can change ingredients without notice.

This 'staple' list includes foods I always try to have on hand. Most foods are non-perishable or if fresh, will be used within a week if you use the weekly menu plan.

Don't be discouraged at how long this takes the first few times around. After a few shopping trips, you will soon become an expert at quickly scanning labels for key ingredients!

I have provided website and ordering information for some of the harder to find foods in the Appendix.

These lists are intended for use after successful implementation of the Induction Diet described in Section 2. Not all of these items are used in the recipes, but having them on hand will allow for flexibility, variation and creativity as you begin your CSID meal and recipe journey.

BEVERAGES

- Welch's Grape Juice - Bottle only
- Dole Pineapple Juice - Canned in 100% juice, not frozen
- Landers 100% pomegranate juice (no other juice added)*
- Distilled water (2 gallons minimum)
- 100% Cranberry juice
- Sparkling mineral water without added sodium*
- Tomato juice* (tomatoes, salt and ascorbic acid only)
- Apple cider (cloudy, not clear)
- Dandelion root tea
- Peppermint tea
- Lemon-ginger tea

FRUITS AND VEGETABLES (FRESH OR FROZEN)

S indicates possible sucrose content
- Green beans (fresh or frozen)
- Fresh or frozen cauliflower
- Grapes (white or red)
- Celery
- Baby carrots ***S***
- Cucumbers
- Lettuce
- Snow peas
- Broccoli
- Kale
- Spinach
- Lettuce (butter, romaine, red leaf, etc.)
- Tomatoes (vine-ripe)
- Avocado
- Strawberries (fresh and frozen, no sugar added)
- Blueberries (fresh or frozen)
- Raspberries
- Lemons (buy in bulk if possible)
- Zucchini (summer squash)
- White mushrooms
- Apples ***S***
- Applesauce ***S***
- Oranges ***S***
- Honey
- Onions ***S***
- Bell peppers (any color)
- Simply fruit jam ***S***
- Ketchup ***S***
- Ranch dressing ***S***
- Mayonnaise ***S***

CANNED/DRY GOODS

- Dry lima beans (or canned butter beans with no additives)

- Canned olives
- Canned pineapple, Dole sweetened with pineapple juice only *S*
- Albacore or yellow fin canned tuna (no broth or soy flakes) in oil or water
- Canned coconut milk with no additives aside from guar gum (boxed is too thin to use with recipes such as crepes)
- Almond butter without added sugar

BAKING AND COOKING INGREDIENTS

- Red wine vinegar
- Dry white wine
- Wheat free tamari
- Cold-pressed olive oil and/or grape seed oil
- Organic coconut oil
- Sea salt
- Pure vanilla extract (check for no-sugar, organic if possible)
- Ener-g baking powder (gluten, wheat, dairy, aluminum free and low sodium) or baking soda
- Individual spices: oregano, basil, thyme, sage, rosemary, dill, black pepper,
- Flax oil
- Unsweetened, finely shredded coconut (order by phone from Lucy's Kitchen Shop or online at nuts.com)
- Flax seed (to grind and add to shakes or baked goods once symptoms have subsided)
- Cinnamon and nutmeg

DAIRY

- Unsalted butter (I add sea salt)
- Whole organic cow's milk
- Heavy whipping cream
- Medium or mild block cheddar cheese
- Block Jack or white cheese
- Plain yogurt (whole milk if you can find it)

- Parmesan cheese* (Fresh Grated with no fillers is best)
- Cottage cheese (only milk, probiotics and stabilizers in the form of vegetable gums)
- Ricotta cheese (only milk, whey, vinegar, xanthium gum stabilizers)
- Cream cheese

MEATS, FISH, POULTRY

- Chicken, (cut-up or whole organic, free-Range if possible)
- Ground/minced turkey
- Ground/minced beef (all natural, grass fed if possible)
- Turkey bacon (use with Sucraid if you cannot find a brand without sugar)
- Fresh water salmon fillet (frozen single portions ok, but check label, Costco Kirkland brand)
- Tilapia fillets
- Fresh sliced turkey or turkey breast strips (glucose added, ok)
- Frozen chicken strips and/or chicken breasts
- Eggs (brown/free range is best) (2 dozen minimum)
- Turkey burgers (Costco, Kirkland Brand are the best!)

FOODS THAT YOU MAY NEED TO ORDER

- Liquid Chlorophyll
- Almond Flour (Lucy's Kitchen Shop or Nuts.com)
- Yogurt Starter (Lucy's Kitchen Shop)

11 - Traveling, School Lunches and More!

Traveling

One of the more challenging aspects we face in managing the CSID diet is being prepared while away from home. Since most meals and ingredients are perishable, traveling becomes a great challenge, especially during the summer. Here are just a few tips that I have found successful over the years.

- Purchase a small, portable ice chest. One of the best investments we ever made, it fits easily in the car, can keep Sucraid cool and makes a great lunch box as well.
- Contact family members and hotels in advance to make sure there will be refrigerated storage space available for you to use upon arrival.
- Buy snack foods in bulk and separate into serving-sized baggies. If you choose to freeze certain foods, you only need to remove enough for one meal at a time. If the serving gets warm, you are only out a small portion. This also makes it easier to grab and go when leaving the hotel or other location for hiking, amusement parks, etc.
- Purchase an emergency medical alert bracelet so that you can show this to personnel at public venues that may not allow you to bring in outside food. Contact the venue in advance to let them know about restricted dietary requirements. Get the name of the on-site manager once you receive approval to bring in food.
- If traveling by airplane, you may have to store Sucraid bottles in checked-in luggage due to safety restrictions. Bring/purchase snacks which will not require Sucraid after passing through security.
- See Snack section under *Soups, Salad, Sides and Snacks* chapter for several ideas.

School Lunches

Perhaps even more challenging than traveling is addressing the issue of school lunches on a daily basis. School lunch menus are packed with high-carbohydrate-based meals and prepared food without easy access to ingredient labels.

School cafeterias are limited as far as preparing separate foods, especially since CSID is not an allergy. Each school site has different regulations, but here is the best approach based on my experience.

1. Prior to the school year beginning, contact the school nurse and cafeteria manager. I have designed a sample "health plan" worksheet at the end of this section to assist you with describing CSID and the dietary limitations. If you have not been able to complete all three phases of the Induction Diet (see Chapter 5), use the Group A worksheet (with or without Sucraid as it applies to your situation.)

2. Ask if the school cafeteria is able to prepare specialty foods. Depending on what is on the menu for the day, preparation may simply mean excluding a bun or sauce with the meal. Samples of food typically stocked and stored for school cafeterias include: string cheese, grilled chicken breasts without breading, plain beef patties, apple slices, grapes, and salad items.

3. If the cafeteria is unable to provide a modified menu, or you are more comfortable providing food, I have provided the quick-reference sample one-week lunch menu below. See referenced recipes section for foods requiring preparation.

Monday
- String cheese
- Sliced, raw zucchini
- 100% grape juice box
- Fruit leather *S*
- Hardboiled egg

Tuesday
- String cheese
- 100% grape juice box
- Apple cookies
- Sliced avocado
- Plain yogurt with berries

Wednesday

- Crepe Wrap (see *Lunch*)
- Sparkling juice (juice and sparkling water only)
- Grape gelatin with whipped cream
- Hardboiled egg

Thursday
- Strawberries and cream cheese
- Celery sticks with almond butter or cream cheese
- Banana Muffin ***S*** (see *Dessert*)
- Cubed, cooked chicken breast
- 100% grape juice box

Friday
- Tuna and Cucumber Salad (see *Lunch*)
- Sliced cheese
- Coconut macaroons (see *Dessert*)
- Sparkling juice (juice and sparkling water only)

Breakfast

The first meal of the day is often packed full of the types of carbohydrates unsuitable for the CSID diet. Rethinking breakfast is a major priority in managing the CSID diet. Though basic, most of these recipes take a bit more time and planning than that quick bowl of cereal or piece of toast.

Almond and Coconut Pancakes

The combination of almond flour and coconut for these pancakes makes them taste more like a gourmet dessert than a healthy breakfast, especially if you top them with whipped cream and blueberries.

Ingredients with an ***S*** to indicate sucrose content.

Yield: 8 pancakes

3 eggs
1/2 cup (125 grams) plain yogurt
1 teaspoon pure vanilla extract
2 tablespoons agave nectar or honey
1/4 teaspoon sea salt
1/2 teaspoon Ener-g baking powder (or 1/4 teaspoon baking soda)
1 cup (100 grams) blanched almond flour
1/2 cup (35 grams) finely shredded unsweetened coconut

Possible Toppings
- Pure Fruit Jam ***S***
- Pure organic maple syrup ***S***
- Mashed blackberries or raspberries ***S***
- Whipped cream made with heavy whipping cream and agave or homemade yogurt and blueberries
- Butter and honey

1. Whisk together eggs, yogurt, and vanilla until creamy. Add agave and salt and mix well.

2. Sift almond flour, baking powder, and coconut into mix. Pour in any larger pieces that won't go through sifter.

3. Melt a teaspoon of coconut oil on low to medium heat on griddle or skillet. Pour pancakes in 1/4 cup portions onto heated griddle.

4. Pancakes must cook slowly in order to cook through without burning. Flip when edges begin to bubble and brown slightly.

5. Serve hot with any of the above-suggested toppings or refrigerate in plastic zipper bags for a take-along snack.

Note on Almonds/Almond Flour

The safe use of almond flour for all CSID phenotypes is undetermined. However, there are many people with other digestive issues such as Crohn's and Celiac that successfully use almonds and almond flour as their flour substitute.

Discuss the possibility with your health practitioner or dietitian to determine if using almond flour is right for your individual situation.

Almond Flour Bread Mini-Loaves

You will want to add this recipe to your list of weekly "batch bake" items. Several recipes call for using almond bread, so having this already baked, cooled and sliced will save you time and give you more freedom in using last-minute recipes calling for almond bread.

Yield: 4 3x6 inch loaves

3 cups blanched almond flour
1/2 teaspoon sea salt
3 teaspoons baking soda
8 eggs
1/4 cup coconut oil, melted
1/4 cup grapeseed or vegetable oil
1/2 teaspoon pure vanilla extract
1/4 cup honey

1. Preheat oven to 350°F. Generously grease mini loaf pans with coconut oil or butter.

2. Sift together almond flour, sea salt and baking powder in a large bowl.

3. Add remaining ingredients and blend well with a wire whisk or electric mixer.

4. Divide batter evenly among bread pans.

5. Bake for 30 minutes or until golden brown and inserted knife comes out clean.

Use for tuna melts, French toast (next page), grilled cheese or any other meal or snack normally calling for traditional bread.

Almond Milk

A great alternative, especially if dairy is off the list. This milk tastes great in cereal or as a replacement for yogurt in smoothies. It can also be used for soups and sauces. The possibilities are endless! Just use wherever you would use normal milk and see what happens!

Yield: 2 quarts milk

3 cups raw almonds, soaked overnight in distilled water
4 or more cups of fresh, distilled water
1/4 cup honey or agave nectar
1/2 teaspoon sea salt

1. Drain and discard the water from the soaked almonds. Pour almonds into a large blender. Add enough fresh distilled water to cover almonds. Blend on high for at least one minute or until liquid is white and frothy.

2. Using doubled cheesecloth or straining cloth, (I use the bag that came with my yogurt maker), line the inside of a 2-quart juice pitcher. Make sure the bag hangs over the outside edge by several inches.

3. Holding the bag in place, slowly pour about half of the almond mixture into the cloth. It will take several minutes to drain.

4. Gently wrap cloth around almond pulp and squeeze additional liquid into the pitcher. Dump almond pulp into a large bowl (use for almond cereal recipe below). Repeat steps 3 and 4 until all almond milk has been filtered.

5. Add honey and salt to almond milk and mix well with a wire whisk. Add more distilled water until you have a full 2 quarts of liquid. Refrigerate and use within 24 hours or freeze.

Almond Cereal

This recipe came from one of my kitchen experiments. I had succeeded in creating a great tasting version of almond milk and was trying to figure out what to do with all the left-over pulp. I didn't want to waste it since almonds are not inexpensive. While trying to make cookies, I was sliding them off the cookie sheet only to have them crumble apart! Annoyed that I had wasted my efforts, I scraped the cookie crumbs into a bowl. I had to laugh when I realized the crumbs looked just like granola!

Yield: 3 cups dry cereal

3 cups almond pulp left over from almond milk (above)
1/2 teaspoon sea salt
1/2 cup honey
1/4 cup butter
2 tablespoons coconut oil
Optional: slivered almonds, coconut flakes, raisins

1. Preheat oven to 300°F.

2. Heat honey, coconut oil, butter and salt in a small pan on low heat, stirring well.

3. Pour honey mixture over almond pulp already in a large bowl. Mix well with a wooden spoon.

4. Spread out almond mixture onto a cookie sheet, smoothing out top with a spatula or your fingers to make sure it is an even thickness.

5. Bake for 1 1/2 to 2 hours, watching carefully that cereal does not burn. Once top layer is a medium golden brown, remove cereal from the oven. Break up pulp and spread evenly on sheet once again. Turn off oven and place cereal back inside, leaving the oven door slightly ajar. (Continued...)

6. Once oven is cool and cereal feels completely dry, pour into a large bowl. Add almond slices, coconut flakes and raisins

as desired. Cereal will keep for about one week in a sealed container or plastic bag. Serve with almond milk, of course!

Bacon, Eggs and Berries Breakfast

Though this is a basic recipe, it is a reminder that even small variations matter while the kinds of foods we offer our children are limited.

Ingredients with an ***S*** to indicates sucrose content.

Yield: about 4 servings

1 pound uncured bacon
sea salt
honey
8 eggs
butter
4 slices almond flour bread
1/2 cup fresh blueberries
1/2 cup fresh raspberries
1 cup fresh strawberries, sliced ***S***
1 cup yogurt

1. Add bacon to a cold non-stick pan. Sprinkle with salt and drizzle with honey. Cook on medium-high heat until crispy.

2. Meanwhile, fry eggs in butter as desired, making sure whites are fully cooked.

3. Spoon 1/4 cup of yogurt on each of four large plates. Top with mixture of berries and drizzle with honey.

4. Place the cooked bacon on paper towels and blot out excess oil with additional paper towels.

5. Add two fried eggs and two slices of bacon to each plate.

6. Serve with Chlorophyll Cocktail, herb tea, or unsweetened almond milk.

Breakfast Quiche

This recipe is a great way to add super foods to breakfast! It also makes a wonderful lunch or snack and tastes even better cold than fresh from the oven.

Yield: 6-8 Servings

Crust
1 cup blanched almond flour
4 tablespoons butter, melted

Filling
1 teaspoon coconut oil
¼ cup (2 ounces) mushrooms, sliced or chopped
4 eggs, beaten
2 tablespoons coconut or almond milk
4 strips cooked, crumbled bacon *S*
1 tomato, sliced
4 ounces shredded cheddar cheese

1. Preheat oven to 325°F.

2. Mix together almond flour and butter and press evenly into bottom and sides of a 9-inch pie dish.

3. Bake the crust for about 10 minutes or until light brown. Place on cooling rack, leaving oven on.

4. Meanwhile, sauté mushrooms in the coconut oil.

5. Add the mushrooms to the pie crust, spreading evenly. Sprinkle bacon on top.

6. Whip together the eggs and coconut milk in a medium bowl. Pour it over the bacon and mushrooms.

7. Gently lay the tomato slices on top of the eggs. Top with grated cheese and bake for 30 minutes or until the eggs are firm and the cheese begins to brown. Serve warm or cold.

Breakfast Crepes

This crepe recipe creates a thicker version of the coconut flour crepes, and is suitable once almond flour has been successfully introduced to the diet. For the unsweetened wrap version, see Lunch chapter.

Yield: 10, 10 inch crepes

6 eggs
1/4 cup blanched almond flour
2 tablespoons coconut flour
1/2 cup coconut milk
2 tablespoons coconut oil
2 tablespoons honey
1 teaspoon pumpkin spice, nutmeg or cinnamon
2 tablespoons freshly ground flax seed (optional after phase 3)
Butter or coconut oil for cooking

1. Combine all ingredients in a blender or food processor aside from the butter for cooking. Blend on high for one minute.

2. Heat a 10-inch skillet on medium-high heat. When a dab of butter sizzles, pan is hot enough.

3. After oiling, pour approximately two tablespoons of batter into skillet, quickly rotating with the handle to coat pan evenly. You may need to experiment with the proper amount as too much or too little will cause the crepe to crumble upon turning.

4. Cook until bubbly and edges cook through. Using a wide spatula, carefully turn crepe over. Cook second side for just a few seconds. Slide crepe onto a cool plate. Repeat.

Filling Variations
- Ricotta cheese and sliced strawberries
- Jam made from pure, low-sucrose fruit such as raspberries or grape
- Plain yogurt and warmed honey

Flour Bread

plain version of quick bread that can be used for ιυα... *)en-faced sandwiches or any other meal normally calling for bread. I admit, the texture takes a little getting used to and I usually add some type of spread such as jam or cream cheese.*

Yield: 1 small loaf

6 eggs
1/2 cup butter, melted
2 tablespoons agave or honey
1/4 teaspoon sea salt
3/4 cup coconut flour
1 teaspoon baking soda

1. Preheat oven to 350°F. Grease inside of small bread pan with coconut oil.

2. Blend all ingredients until smooth.

3. Pour into prepared bread pan. Bake for 40 minutes.

4. Cool completely. Cut into thin slices.

Use for French toast, tuna melts, breakfast toast, grilled cheese sandwiches and more.

Coconut Flour Crepes

These pancakes have the taste and texture of the crepes my mother used to make, but without the white flour. They can be used as substitute tortillas for tacos, quesadillas or sandwich wraps. It is best to use two crepes together since they tend to crumble easily.

Ingredients with an ***S*** to indicates sucrose content.

Yield: 8 6-inch crepes

4 eggs
2 tablespoons coconut oil, melted
1/2 teaspoon pure vanilla extract
1/3 cup coconut milk from can (without added sugars or starches) or heavy whipping cream
1 teaspoon agave or honey
sea salt
2 tablespoons coconut flour
Fresh blueberries, raspberries, or strawberries (***S*** -maybe)
Sour cream or plain yogurt (optional)

1. Blend eggs, coconut oil, vanilla, coconut milk, agave, salt and coconut flour in blender or food processor until smooth.

2. Melt 1 teaspoon butter in a small skillet on medium heat. Pour about 2 tablespoons batter into heated pan, turning pan to spread batter into a thin circle. (Too much batter will cause the crepe to crumble when you try to flip it- if you pour too much, you will have to cook longer to be able to flip it.) When edges begin to bubble and turn golden brown, flip over carefully. Cook second side for just a few seconds and slide crepe onto a large plate.

3. Spread about 1 teaspoon of sour cream and a few mashed berries on crepe. Roll. Serve with warmed drizzled honey if desired.

Organic Coconut Oil

There are entire books devoted to explaining the many benefits of incorporating coconut oil into a regular diet. See the Bibliography for a list of titles.

To summarize, coconut oil helps the body to fight off free radicals, requires less enzymes from our body in order to break it downs, improves absorption of vitamins and minerals, is known to sooth and heal inflammation and injury to the digestive tract, and contains antimicrobial fats that can fight off germs and parasites. And that is a very short list only highlighting the benefits for the digestive system.

I use coconut oil to cook anything on the stove from sautéing vegetables to cooking chicken and eggs. I grease pans with it for baking, add it to smoothies, and use it instead of butter for a variety of baked goods and desserts.

French Toast with Berries and Cinnamon Eggs

This rich and filling breakfast makes a great Saturday morning brunch. Slice bread thin to make this stretch for up to 3 servings.

Yield: 2 servings

1 loaf mini almond bread
3 large eggs
2 tablespoons milk (any variety-- cows, goats, soy, coconut or almond without added sugars)
1 teaspoon pure vanilla extract
1/4 teaspoon cinnamon
1/2 cup fresh strawberries, sliced
1/4 cup honey, warmed
Butter or coconut oil for cooking

1. Slice off top and bottom of almond bread loaf. Slicing along the length, make 4-6 pieces.

2. Mix eggs, milk, vanilla and cinnamon until well blended.

3. Place one to two slices of bread into egg mixture and allow soaking for at least one minute on each side. Meanwhile, preheat skillet to medium-high heat.

4. Melt butter or coconut oil in skillet. Add egg-soaked almond bread slices and cook until both sides are golden brown.

5. Remove from heat and top with strawberries and honey.

6. Cook remaining egg batter for side of cinnamon eggs. You may wish to add another egg depending on how many servings you are producing.

3. Pour honey mixture over almond pulp already in a large bowl. Mix well with a wooden spoon.

4. Spread out almond mixture onto a cookie sheet, smoothing out top with a spatula or your fingers to make sure it is an even thickness.

Rainbow Scrambled Eggs

Start the morning right with a balanced combination of proteins and vegetables.

Yield: 2 servings

4 eggs
1 tablespoon butter
2 fresh, small mushrooms, sliced or chopped
1/2 cup chopped blend of red, orange and yellow bell pepper
S
1/4 cup fresh or steamed broccoli crowns, kale, or spinach; finely chopped
1/2 tomato, chopped
1 tablespoon sour cream, starch-free (no maltodextrin) variety (optional)
Sea salt and pepper to taste

1. Whisk together the eggs and in a small bowl.

2. Sauté butter and mushrooms on medium heat for about one minute.

3. Add eggs and broccoli, stirring constantly with spatula until eggs are cooked through.

4. Place eggs onto plate and add salt, pepper, tomatoes, and sour cream as desired.

Rise and Shine Smoothie

When there is no time for cooking crepes, pancakes or eggs, this smoothie can be the fast breakfast without compromising healthy. If bananas are not tolerable at this point, simply omit them and add a little ice to keep the thick texture.

Yield: 16 ounces, or 4 servings

1/2 cup frozen blueberries or strawberries
1 ripe banana (brown spots, no green on peel) ***S***
1/2 cup plain yogurt
2 tablespoons honey or agave
Recommended dose of powdered vitamins
1 tablespoon flax oil
1 tablespoon coconut oil
1 tablespoon liquid chlorophyll (optional)

Blend all ingredients until smooth. Serve cold with a fun straw.

Lunch

If your child is in school, lunch may also prove
to be a difficult meal to adjust to. See the
appendix for a sample form to assist you with
communicating your child's diet restrictions at
school. For many of these recipes, I double
them and store in single size servings. The
second meal of the day is also a great
opportunity to use up leftovers from dinner.
Many of these meals are also simple enough
that you can have your older children make
them on their own, or allow younger children to
assist you.

Crepe Wraps

This unsweetened version of breakfast crepes can substitute tortillas or wraps for a great to-go lunch option. Batch bake with Breakfast Crepes to have plenty of breakfast and lunch options for the week.

Yield: 10, 10 inch crepes

6 eggs
1/4 cup blanched almond flour
2 tablespoons coconut flour
1/2 cup coconut milk
2 tablespoons coconut oil
1/8 teaspoon sea salt
Butter or coconut oil for cooking

1. Combine all ingredients in a blender or food processor aside from the butter for cooking. Blend on high for one minute.

2. Heat a 10-inch skillet on medium-high heat. When a dab of butter sizzles, pan is hot enough.

3. Pour approximately two tablespoons of batter into pan, quickly rotating with the handle to coat pan evenly. You may need to experiment with the proper amount as too much or too little will cause the crepe to crumble upon turning.

4. Cook until bubbly and edges cook through. Using a wide spatula, carefully turn crepe over. Cook second side for just a few seconds. Slide crepe onto a cool plate. Repeat.

Filling Variations-Wraps
- Baby spinach, cream cheese and strawberry slices
- Sliced turkey breast, cream cheese and cranberry/orange sauce
- Tuna mixed with sour cream or plain yogurt and thinly sliced cucumber

.cks with Almond Butter

cipe makes a great snack or take-along addition to any lunch. Or pre slice celery and store in a plastic container in the refrigerator alongside the almond butter for a quick boost of protein and fiber any time of day.

Yield: 2 servings

4 celery stalks, sliced into 2-inch long sticks
1/4 cup fresh ground almond butter
honey (optional)

1. Spread 1 teaspoon of almond butter on each celery stick.

2. Drizzle with honey.

3. Serve immediately or cover with plastic wrap and refrigerate for up to 2 days.

Variations
- Substitute Almond butter for cream cheese for Group A and add sliced red grapes
- Group B (some starch allowed) may also add raisins

Cucumber, Cheese and Turkey Sandwiches

Most lunches for this menu will contain a combination of snack-like foods and leftovers. These mini sandwiches make a great in between meal snack. You can also pack ingredients separately and store them in a small ice-chest for an on-the go snack.

Yield: 2 servings

1 medium cucumber (about 8-inches in length), peeled and cut into 16 slices
2 4-inch slices of medium cheddar cheese cut into quarters (making 8 small slices total)
2 slices of oven-roasted turkey breast (no added starch or sugar), cut into quarters (making 8 small slices total)

1. Lay eight of the cucumber slices flat on a large plate. Layer one slice of cheese and once slice of turkey on top of each cucumber slice and top with remaining cucumber.

2. Serve with red grapes on the side.

Tuna and Cucumber Salad Served on Cheese Slices

You may choose to cut up or grate cheese on top and serve this salad in a bowl depending on individual preferences. My son didn't care for the cheese, and just ate it from a bowl.

Yield: 3 cups or 6 servings

2 can albacore tuna, drained
1/2 cup plain yogurt
Juice from 1/2 a lemon
1 teaspoon salt
2 cucumbers, peeled and cubed
6 thick slices of cheddar or Colby cheese

1. Combine tuna, yogurt and lemon until tuna is mashed well and moist.

2. A cucumbers and salt to taste.

3. Scoop onto cheese slices.

Tuna Melts with Avocado and Tomato

These are a great source of protein, fiber and omega 3 oils. Group C can also use sprouted grain bread if desired.

Yield: 2 servings

1 (6-ounce) can Albacore tuna (no soy or broth added)
2 tablespoons plain yogurt
1 garden fresh tomato, sliced
4 slices cheddar cheese
1 avocado, sliced
2 crepe wraps, 2 slices coconut bread or 2 slices almond bread

1. Preheat oven to 425°F or use foil covered tray in the toaster oven.

2. Drain water from tuna can, and scoop tuna into a small bowl. Add the yogurt and mix well.

3. Lightly toast almond bread and place slices side by side on a lightly buttered cookie sheet. If using coconut crepes fold crepes in half and do not reheat.

4. Divide tuna into equal portions and spread onto the toasted bread. Top with a slice each of cheese and tomato.

5. Bake for 10 to 15 minutes or until cheese is melted. Add sliced avocado. Serve.

Turkey Patty with Tomato and Cheese

Think of your ground turkey patty without the bun as you would a slice of turkey fresh from the bird. You won't miss the bread with the yummy combination of Jack cheese and garden fresh tomato.

Yield: 1 serving

1 ground turkey patty (make your own with ground turkey or use any brand of pre-packaged 100% turkey patty that does not include added sugar or starches)
1 slice Jack cheese
1 slice garden fresh tomato
Avocado (optional)

1. Heat up a small frying pan on medium heat. Use a small amount of olive oil if desired.

2. Place turkey patty on hot oil, cooking thoroughly on both sides.

3. Remove from heat and top with cheese, tomato and avocado as desired.

Serve with steamed, organic green beans, fresh spinach salad topped with sunflower seeds, currants and lemon juice.

Soups, Salads, Sides and Snacks

Chicken and Lima Bean Soup

You will need to plan ahead for this recipe by soaking and cooking the beans the night before. If you choose to use canned butter beans, be sure to read the label, drain well and add distilled water to reduce sodium. Then combine ingredients as directed and refrigerate until about 30 minutes before the meal to allow time to reheat. You may also cook and divide in single-sized servings in freezer bags ahead of time. Boil bags to reheat and serve with fresh baked, buttered almond bread and a garden salad.

Ingredients with an ***S*** to indicates sucrose content.

Yield: 12, 1 cup servings

1/2 yellow onion, chopped ***S***
2 celery stalks, chopped
1 tablespoon olive oil
1 teaspoon dried oregano
1 teaspoon dried thyme
1 teaspoon dried rosemary
1 pound Lima beans, soaked and boiled (or 2 cans butter beans, drained)
2 cups cooked and cubed chicken breast
1 whole tomato, diced
2 organic carrots, peeled and chopped
Sea salt and Pepper to taste

1. Using a 4-quart pot, sauté onions and celery in olive oil in large pot with olive oil on medium-high heat for about 2-minutes.

2. Stir in oregano, thyme, and rosemary and cook for about a minute to release oils.

3. Add beans, chicken, tomato, carrots and enough water to cover ingredients by about a half an inch.

4. Reduce heat to low and simmer for 45 minutes to an hour, adding sea salt and pepper to taste.

5. If you plan to batch and store the soup, pour into containers and cool completely before covering and freezing. To reheat, place storage container in a shallow pan of water and heat on low.

6. Add tomato juice if soup consistency is too thick

Sea Salt

Sea salt has the opposite effect on the body as iodized or regular salt. Salt is an essential part of the healthy function of the body. In its natural state, the sodium in salt assists in the digestive process and works with other nutrients to balance out the body's pH levels.

Regular table salt, in its refined state actually causes more stress on the body – hence resulting in the opposite, acidic affect.

I use sea salt to re-season canned beans and vegetables after draining and rinsing off salt water from manufacturing.

Green Beans in Mushroom Sauce

I made this recipe for my contribution to Thanksgiving dinner this past fall. All of the adults, including my daughter with CSID, absolutely loved them! They will be on our list of traditional Holiday recipes from now on.

Ingredients with an ***S*** to indicates sucrose content.

Yield: 8 servings

3 cups fresh green beans, steamed until bright green
1/4 cup butter
1 small yellow onion, finely chopped ***S***
1 pound fresh mushrooms, sliced and chopped
1/4 cup dry white wine (optional) ***S***
2 teaspoons sea salt
1 quart heavy whipping cream

1. Sauté onion in on medium-high heat in 2 tablespoons of butter until translucent. Add mushrooms and sauté until mushrooms begin to brown.

2. Add wine and salt. Cook for five minutes and reduce heat to medium-low.

3. Add whipping cream, and simmer for about 20 minutes, stirring occasionally until sauce thickens.

4. Meanwhile, preheat oven to 350°F and grease a large casserole dish generously with remaining butter.

5. Place steamed green beans into casserole dish. Pour mushroom cream sauce over green beans.

6. Bake until bubbly. Top with sliced almond and grated parmesan cheese if desired. Serve.

Green Salad with Tomatoes and Shredded Carrots

This salad makes a great addition to an otherwise meat-filled meal. You will get plenty of vital enzymes and leafy greens to help bring pH balance to your overall meal. The use of a purely lemon juice dressing also assists digestion.

Yield: 4 servings

4 large organic Romaine lettuce leaves, washed and torn into bite-size pieces
4 ounces organic baby spinach
4 organic green lettuce leaves, washed and torn into bite-sized pieces
1 cup alfalfa sprouts
2 fresh, organic meat tomatoes, sliced
2 organic carrots, grated or shredded in food processor
Juice from 1 lemon

1. Mix together lettuce and carrots and place in large bowl.

2. Spread sprouts out evenly over lettuce and carrots.

3. Top with tomatoes.

4. Add lemon juice and serve immediately.

Mashed Cauliflower (Fake Potatoes!)

For best results, serve this in a bowl, as it tends to turn out a bit runnier than traditional potatoes. However, the taste of these fake potatoes trumps consistency any day. This side dish goes well with pork chops, turkey meat loaf, or grilled chicken breasts.

Yield: 8 servings

2 fresh cauliflower crowns
2-4 tablespoons butter (to taste)
1/4 cup (more or less) heavy whipping cream
Real Salt or sea salt and pepper to taste

1. Boil cauliflower in a large pot until you can easily slice a fork through the crowns. Drain.
2. Combine butter, whipping cream and cauliflower in mixing bowl. Using electric beaters, mix on medium speed until creamy.
4. Add salt, pepper, and serve warm with additional butter, or gravy (recipe on next page).

Gravy (optional)

Yield: about 6 ounces

2 tablespoons meat drippings
1/2 cup water
1 tablespoons wheat free tamari sauce
Real Salt and pepper to taste
2 tablespoons Thick 'N Thin Not Starch (order online at www.expertfoods.com)

1. Whisk all ingredients together in a small pan on medium-low heat.

2. Stir constantly until thick and smooth. Serve immediately or batch and freeze for later use.

Spinach and Strawberry Salad

This simple salad combination makes a great addition to any lunch or dinner plate.

Yield: 4 servings

1 bag prewashed baby spinach
1 quart fresh strawberries, sliced
Almond slices (optional)

Toss all ingredients. Serve with a bit of lemon juice if desired.

Sweet 'N Crunchy Salad

This sweet and crunchy salad makes a great cool side dish or snack. It will keep in the refrigerator for up to 24 hours, but don't be surprised if it is gone way before that!

Ingredients with an ***S*** to indicates sucrose content.

Yield: 10, 1/2 cup servings

3 stalks celery, finely chopped
2 medium apples peeled and chopped ***S***
1 cup halved or quartered red grapes
1/4 cup slivered, blanched almonds (optional)
1/2 cup plain or homemade yogurt
Honey or agave to taste
1/4 cup raisins (optional-Group C only)

1. Place all of the ingredients except for the yogurt in a medium-sized bowl, and stir to mix well. Add the yogurt, and stir just until the ingredients are well coated.

2. Serve the salad in half-cup portions.

Snacks

These are not really recipes, just ideas for different food combinations and quick foods to have on hand whenever possible. Many of these can be used for school lunches or road trips as well.

Ingredients with an ***S*** to indicates sucrose content.

- Hard boiled eggs
- Red or white grapes
- Sliced cheese or string cheese
- Almond flour muffins or cookies (See recipes in Desserts section)
- Sliced cucumbers, celery, bell peppers ***S***, carrots
- Apples ***S*** and/or celery and almond butter
- Dry almond cereal as a trail mix
- Coconut Macaroons
- Sweet mini-peppers
- Cottage cheese (check ingredients) with sliced ripe bananas ***S*** and honey
- Peeled and sliced raw zucchini spears
- Cooked, cubed chicken breasts
- Zucchini (green summer squash), raw and sliced
- Homemade or fruit-juice sweetened dried fruit leather (apple, strawberry, grape, raspberry)

Dinner

Most of these meals were designed to feed your whole family. If you have been making separate meals for your CSID child, using these meals to feed everyone will hopefully bring you some relief.

Bone-In Pork Roast

This makes a great Sunday dinner. Just prepare as directed around lunch time and take some time to revive yourself for the coming week, while dinner cooks itself! Limit overall servings of pork I have heard from several sources that it creates stress on the digestive system to break down. Also, pork generally contains high levels of toxins due to the way pigs are raised and farmed in America.

Yield: 8 to 10 servings

1 bone-in pork roast (fresh, unseasoned)
4 garlic cloves, pressed (optional)
1 tablespoon sea salt
1 teaspoon black pepper
2 tablespoons wheat free tamari sauce
1 pound fresh, organic baby carrots ***S***

1. Place the pork roast in a large crock-pot. Make a slit across the top about an inch deep.

2. Insert the garlic cloves into the slit and sprinkle top with salt and pepper. Pour Tamari sauce over top, making sure it soaks into the slit with the garlic. Place raw carrots around sides of roast.

3. Cover and cook on low for 5-6 hours.

5. Slice and serve roast with Mashed Cauliflower and Gravy made with juices from the roast.

Cranberry Orange Chicken with Dill

This is yet again, another recipe I made out of necessity with what I already had in my refrigerator. This recipe can still be enjoyed without including orange juice if Sucraid is not available. To enjoy this recipe year-round, be sure to purchase and freeze several bags of fresh cranberries every fall.

Yield: 4 to 6 servings

1 12-ounce bag fresh cranberries (I usually buy extra bags during the holidays and freeze them for later use, as cranberries are only available seasonally)
Juice of one freshly squeezed orange ***S***
1/2 cup agave or honey
2 pounds of chicken leg quarters, thawed OR 8-10 individually frozen chicken tenders
1 cup water
1 teaspoon dried dill weed
Sea salt and pepper to taste

1. Place cranberries, water, orange juice and sweetener in medium sauce pan on medium/high heat until boiling.

2. Simmer about 30 minutes or until cranberries are soft and smash down easily.

3. Place in refrigerator for 1 hour.

4. Place chicken in a large Crockpot and rub skin with salt and pepper.

5. Pour cranberry/orange mixture over chicken.

6. Cook on Low for 6 to 7 hours.

STOVE-TOP Alternative
1. Melt 2 tablespoons butter in a large frying pan on medium-high heat.

2. Cook leg quarters or chicken tenders until golden brown and cooked thoroughly. Set aside on a large serving platter.

3. Add cranberries, water, orange juice and honey to frying pan used for chicken. Bring to boil, stirring often.

4. Reduce heat and simmer for 15 minutes or until cranberries pop and liquid begins to thicken.

5. Pour cranberry mixture over chicken. Sprinkle with dill and serve.

Creamy Chicken Casserole

This recipe mocks the traditional chicken and cream of mushroom recipe, replacing rice with zucchini and using a homemade creamy mushroom sauce that is not only starch-free but far more flavorful.

Yield: 8 servings

2 tablespoons butter
4 cups zucchini, sliced into 1/4 inch or less in thickness
2 cups chicken breast, cooked and cubed
1 cup mushrooms, coarsely chopped
1/2 cup yellow onion, finely chopped ***S*** (optional)
1/2 cup sour cream
2 teaspoons sea salt
2 teaspoons black pepper
2 cups cheddar cheese, shredded

1. Preheat oven to 425°F. Coat a large casserole dish with butter, covering inside edges and corners well.

2. Sauté mushrooms and onion in butter until onions are clear.

2. Stack zucchini slices evenly along bottom of the dish. Layer chicken on top of zucchini.

3. Blend sautéed mushrooms and onion, sour cream, salt, and pepper in food processor until smooth and creamy. Spread on top of the chicken.

4. Cover with foil and bake for 30 minutes. Remove foil and add cheese. Bake an additional 10 minutes or until cheese is melted.

Deep Dish Layered Pizza with Almond Flour Crust

Serve this juicy pizza in bowls and top with sour cream.

Yield: 8 to 10 servings

Topping
2 pounds ground beef
1 teaspoon dried oregano
1 teaspoon dried thyme
1 small or 1/2 medium onion, thinly sliced ***S***
3 cups tomato juice
1/4 cup red wine vinegar
1/2 teaspoon sea salt
1- 6 oz. can black olives, sliced
4 ounces cheddar cheese, grated
1/2 cup mushrooms, coarsely chopped
1 small zucchini, coarsely chopped

Almond Flour Crust
1/2 cup blanched almond flour
1 egg
1/4 teaspoon sea salt
1 tablespoon olive oil

1. Sauté ground beef over medium-high heat in a large skillet until brown. Drain off excess fat and add oregano, thyme, and onion. Stir for one minute, allowing oils from spices to resonate and onion to turn clear. Reduce heat.

2. Add the tomato juice, vinegar, salt and olives, and simmer. Preheat oven to 425°F.

3. Meanwhile, mix together almond flour, egg, and salt.

4. Pour half a tablespoon of the olive oil into a large pie pan and spread the almond crust mixture evenly along bottom and sides of dish. Bake the crust for 10 minutes or until the top begins to brown.

5. Remove the crust from the oven and reduce oven temperature to 400°F. Spread half of the beef mixture over

the crust. Layer half of the cheese over the beef and then add all of the mushrooms and zucchini on top of the cheese.

6. Add the rest of the hamburger mixture and top with the remaining cheese.

7. Bake pizza uncovered for 40 minutes or until cheese is bubbly and begins to brown.

Fried Chicken Patties

Miniature, ground chicken patties add amazing flavor to any tomato sauce. Add them to the Tomato-Basil sauce and serve over spaghetti sauce with parmesan cheese.

Yield: 30 1-inch rounds

1 egg
1/4 cup blanched almond flour
1/2 cup yellow onion, finely chopped ***S***
1/2 red bell pepper, chopped ***S***
1/4 teaspoon sea salt
1 pound natural ground chicken
3-5 tablespoons cold-pressed, virgin olive oil

1. In a medium-sized bowl, mix egg, almond flour, onion, bell pepper, and salt with a wire whisk until well blended. Add chicken and mix well.

2. Using a large pan on medium-high heat, add one tablespoon of olive oil. Scoop out 1/4 cup chicken mixture and place on heated pan, smashing down to form a patty-sized disk.

3. Cook for approximately three minutes on each side, or until brown and crispy. For best results, use metal tongs to turn patties.

4. Serve topped with tomato sauce or serve alone with spaghetti squash and a garden salad.

Ground Turkey with Zucchini and Carrots

We were planning on staying with friends on New Year's Eve and I knew there would be plenty of off-limits food available throughout the night. I haphazardly threw together whatever I had in the fridge in an effort to have something healthy available for my family and anyone else not wanting to indulge in the typical snack food well into the night. Not only did everyone at the party love it, my friend asked for the recipe!

Yield: 6 servings

1 pound unseasoned ground turkey
36 ounces tomato juice
3 medium, organic zucchini, in ¼ inch slices
3 large, organic carrots
sea salt) & pepper to taste

1. Cook turkey on medium-high heat until done. Drain excess fat.

2. Add tomato sauce, zucchini, carrots, salt and pepper. Reduce heat to medium-low.

3. Simmer for one hour, stirring occasionally. Serve hot and top with freshly grated parmesan cheese if desired.

Hawaiian Pizza with Cauliflower Crust

Having a pizza alternative works well for birthdays or Friday night-in. Making the sauce (step 5) and steaming and cooling the cauliflower in advance will cut preparation time in half. The crust isn't quite as firm as flour-based crust, so be ready to use a fork and dig in!

Yield: 8 servings

Cauliflower Crust
2 tablespoons/30 ml olive oil
4 cups/1 liter boiled cauliflower crowns, steamed and cooled*
2 eggs
1 cup/280 grams grated mozzarella cheese (do not buy pre-grated as potato starch is added)

Pizza Topping
16 ounces/500 ml tomato juice
Real Salt and black pepper to taste
1 cup grated mozzarella cheese
4 ounces ham** (check label for no sugar or starch fillers added; dextrose is okay) ***S***
4 ounces pineapple slices (in 100% pineapple juice if using canned) ***S***

**Hormel® black label ham does not add starches and only adds dextrose.

1. Preheat oven to 450°F.

2. Coat pie dish with 1 tablespoon olive oil. I used an IKEA pie plate with removable bottom.

3. Combine cauliflower, cheese and egg in food processor and blend until smooth. A few small bits of cauliflower will remain.

4. Spread cauliflower mixture evenly in pie dish. Bake crust for 12-15 minutes or until settled and light brown. If using a

pie plate with removable bottom, you may want to place on a cookie sheet to catch drips.

5. Meanwhile, combine the tomato juice with the salt and pepper in a small saucepan and cook on medium high until it thickens to the consistency of tomato sauce.

7. Remove the crust from the oven and drizzle remaining olive oil on top.

8. Spread the tomato sauce mix on the crust. Add remaining cheese, ham and pineapple.

9. Bake for 10 to 12 minutes or until the cheese is melted and begins to bubble.

10. Cool for at least 5 minutes. Slice carefully and serve on a plate with a fork.

Variations
- Replace ham and pineapple with turkey pepperoni that does not contain added sugar or starch.
- Replace ham and pineapple with thinly sliced mushrooms and zucchini for a vegetarian version.
- Replace mozzarella cheese with jack cheese to reduce lactose.

Salmon Fillets with Dill and Lemon

Serve this simple meal at least once per week to fulfill part of the three servings of fish needed for complete nutrition.

Yield: 6 servings

4 to 6 individually wrapped, 2-ounce salmon fillets, boneless, skinless
Juice from one whole, fresh lemon
2 teaspoons dry dill weed
4 tablespoons butter

1. Preheat oven to 425°F. Butter a 9x12 inch baking dish.

2. Place salmon fillets in dish, evenly spaced.

3. Pour lemon juice over fillets. Sprinkle dill weed evenly over fillets.

4. Top each fillet with 1/2 tablespoon butter

5. Cover with foil and bake for 20 to 25 minutes or until salmon flakes easily with a fork.

6. Serve with sautéed fresh green beans and a salad.

Spaghetti Squash & Sauce

You will find it easy to transition to this starch-free substitute for spaghetti. In addition, you have many more topping choices than with noodles from a sweet honey and butter treat to traditional tomato sauce.

Yield: 4 to 6 servings depending on the size of the squash

Tomato Basil Sauce
2 tablespoons olive oil
5 medium mushrooms, sliced
1 64-ounce bottle 100% tomato juice (tomatoes, salt and vitamin C only)
6-8 peeled, fresh garden beefsteak tomatoes
12 ounces fresh, organic basil
black pepper

1 medium spaghetti squash

Preheat oven to 375°F.

1. Carefully cut the squash in half, lengthwise and do not remove seeds. If this is too difficult due to the hard outer shell, you may want to boil the squash whole for about 10 minutes in a large pot until the shell softens a bit.

2. Place both pieces, cut-side down into a large casserole dish. Pour water into the dish to about one-inch in depth.

4. Bake for about 1 hour depending on the size of the squash. Remove carefully and allow several minutes for cooling.

5. Meanwhile, sauté the mushrooms with olive oil in a 2–quart pot until mushrooms brown.

6. Blend 1 cup tomato juice, peeled tomatoes, and basil leaves until smooth. Add tomato and basil mixture to the mushroom.

7. Stir in remaining tomato juice and cook on medium-high heat until boiling. Turn down to low heat. Simmer for at least 30 minutes, stirring occasionally and adding pepper to taste.

8. Once squash has cooled slightly, carefully turn each squash side over, using oven mitts if needed. Scoop out squash into a bowl with a fork and discard the seeds.

9. Add cooked, seeded spaghetti squash to sauce and toss. Serve with butter and parmesan cheese if desired.

Additional Topping Options

- Grated cheddar cheese
- Honey, butter & cinnamon
- Add 1 pound cooked, ground turkey to step 5 if desired

Turkey Meat Loaf

You won't miss a thing with this juicy, low-fat and starch-free version of the traditional recipe. Serve with mashed cauliflower, steamed zucchini and a garden salad.

Yield: 8 servings

2 pounds ground turkey
2 eggs, slightly beaten
1/4 cup cooked butter beans, mashed and drained or ¼ cup blanched almond flour
1 teaspoon sea salt
1/2 teaspoon black pepper
2 teaspoons red wine vinegar
1/3 cup tomato juice (tomatoes, salt and vitamin C only)
½ small yellow onion, finely chopped ***S***

1. Preheat oven to 425°F.

2. Combine all ingredients in a large bowl, and mix well using a wooden spoon.

3. Pour into a full-sized loaf pan. Place pan on cookie sheet to catch drips and bake for 1 hour or until thermometer inserted in center reads at least 180°F.

4. If serving with ketchup, Sucraid is needed.

Zucchini Lasagna

This is one of those meals where zucchini is easily disguised as pasta. It is extremely juicy and often calls for a second helping!

Yield: 8 servings

1 pound ground turkey
4 cups mushrooms, finely chopped
1 teaspoon dried oregano
1 teaspoon dried basil
1 teaspoon dried thyme
¼ cup red wine vinegar
4 ounces hard, white cheese, grated
4 ounces cheddar cheese, grated
1/2 cup Parmesan cheese, grated
2 cups 100% tomato juice *(nothing aside from tomato juice from concentrate, salt and vitamin C as ascorbic acid)*
sea salt and black pepper to taste

6 medium zucchini peeled and sliced lengthwise into 4 to 6 slices each *(Spread out slices on platters and sprinkle with salt to release excess water. Dab off water   with   paper towel before layering in lasagna dish)*

1. In a large pot on medium heat, brown the ground turkey. Drain the fat, leaving a tablespoon or so for sautéing.

2. Add the mushrooms, oregano, basil, thyme to the pan used for cooking the ground turkey. Sauté until mushroom are soft.

3. Stir in the tomato juice and season with salt and pepper. Simmer for 15 minutes or until sauce thickens.

4. Preheat the oven to 450°F. Cover a 9- X 13- inch casserole dish with butter and layer about one third of the zucchini slices. Pour one third of the meat sauce on top of the zucchini. Sprinkle one third of the grated cheese over sauce.

6. Repeat the layers two more times and sprinkle Parmesan cheese over the top.

7. Bake for 45 minutes to 1 hour, until it is bubbly and the cheese on top is crispy and browned to your liking.

8. Remove from the oven and let sit for 5 minutes before serving.

9. Cut the lasagna and use a slotted spatula to serve it.

Zucchini produces a lot of liquid when it cooks, and the slotted utensil allows the excess water to drain off.

Beverages

Roanne King

Blueberry Smoothie

Kids won't even know they are getting vital nutrients as they sip or spoon this cool, blue treat in addition to lunch or as dessert on a hot summer evening.

Yield: 4 servings

1/2 cup whole organic milk, coconut milk, or almond milk*
1/2 cup frozen blueberries
1/2 cup whole plain yogurt
1 tablespoon coconut oil
1 tablespoon flax oil
1 tablespoon honey or agave

1. Blend blueberries with the milk until smooth, adding more milk if needed.

2. Add remaining ingredients and blend on high until frothy. Serve immediately.

Chlorophyll Cocktail

My husband named this drink a cocktail because of its numerous ingredients. However, contrary to a typical 'cocktail', this beverage is alcohol free!

Yield: 2 servings

1/2 fresh-squeezed lemon
2 teaspoons Nature's Sunshine Liquid Chlorophyll
4 ounces distilled water
1/2 teaspoon L-glutamine powder
1 teaspoon flax oil
2 teaspoons agave or honey

1. Mix all of the ingredients well and divide into two 4-ounce cups or containers.

2. Cocktail should be taken with any meals containing meats, eggs, or cheese to assist in digestion or as a between-meal supplement to boost blood sugar and increase calories.

Lemon-Lime Sparkling Slushy

A twist on the standard lemon-lime homemade soda, you may simply omit blending the ice with other ingredients to convert this to a traditionally flavored drink.

Yield: 1-2 Servings

8 ounces (236ml) sparkling, sodium-free mineral water
4 ounces (250 ml) ice
1 fresh lemon
1 fresh lime
2 tablespoons honey, or agave

1. Add all ingredients to blender and blend until frothy.

2. Serve immediately.

No Banana Smoothie

Use this recipe if you are not comfortable with introducing bananas to the diet or if you do not have any ripe bananas.

Yield: 4 to 6 servings

1/2 cup homemade yogurt
2 tablespoons organic, cold-pressed coconut oil
2 tablespoons flax oil
½ cup fresh squeezed orange juice (not from concentrate)
S
2 tablespoons agave or honey
1/4 cup almond flour
1/2 cup fresh or frozen blueberries, raspberries or strawberries
Liquid or powdered vitamins
Ice for desired consistency

1. Blend yogurt, agave, oils, and orange juice until smooth.

2. While blender is running, slowly add the berries and then almond flour. If you use fresh berries, smoothie will have a liquid consistency.

3. Add ice to reach desired consistency and serve immediately.

Pomegranate Juice with a Boost

This icy drink contains antioxidants, omega-3 oils, and healing aloe to help sooth damaged digestive systems. Make and serve as directed, or blend together all ingredients, pour into ice-cube trays and add to Welch's grape juice for an extra boost of nutrients and flavor.

Yield: 3 servings

1/2 cup crushed ice
1/2 cup 100% pomegranate juice
1 tablespoon flax oil
1 tablespoon pure liquid aloe-vera juice
2 teaspoons agave
1 dropper liquid vitamins (or as prescribed by doctor)
1/2 cup of distilled, purified, or sparkling mineral water

1. Add ice and pomegranate juice to a one-quart or larger pitcher and stir.

2. Add remaining ingredients, stirring until agave is dissolved

3. Pour into 4 ounce cups, inserting colorful bendy straws if desired and serve immediately.

Raspberry-Mint Delight

Refreshing and only slightly sweet, this beverage makes a wonderful summer-afternoon treat. Blend with ice for a slushy, frothy result!

Yield: About 2 quarts

6 peppermint tea bags
1 cup (250 ml) boiled water
1/4 cup honey or agave nectar
12 ounces (240 grams) fresh or frozen raspberries
6 cups or 1.5 liters cold water
2 cups (500 ml) ice (if making a slushy)

1. Steep tea bags in boiled water for ten minutes.

2. Add honey or agave and mix until dissolved.

3. Blend raspberries in about 3 cups of the cold water and ice if desired.

4. Pour blended raspberries, tea and remaining cold water into a large pitcher or tea jar.

5. Serve with ice if you didn't already blend it on step 3 or refrigerate.

6. Garnish with fresh mint leaves and colorful straws and serve.

Special Grape-Apple Soda

It is no fun watching your child watch other children eating or drinking something they can't. When I discovered a way to make special soda, the tables soon turned and all of Parker's siblings wanted some of their own. It's fast and easy enough for school-aged children to prepare for themselves.

Yield: 2-4 servings

4 ounces (250 ml) 100% grape juice
4 ounces (250 ml) fresh pressed apple cider
8 ounces (500 ml) sparkling, sodium-free mineral water
2 ounces honey or agave

1. Pour all ingredients into a large pitcher.

2. Mix with a spoon until sweetener is dissolved.

3. Serve with ice if desired.

Variations
Use 8 total ounces of one kind of juice. 100% pomegranate or 100% cranberry juices are also acceptable.

Roanne King

Dessert

Upside-Down Pineapple & Coconut Muffins

These muffins are extremely sweet and moist. Eat them as they are or slice them in half and spread on a dollop of butter.

Yield: 12 muffins

4 tablespoons butter, melted
1/3 cup honey
1/2 cup plain yogurt
3 eggs, beaten
1/2 cup unsweetened shredded coconut
2 cups blanched almond flour
1/2 teaspoon baking soda
1/4 teaspoon sea salt
1 cup crushed pineapple (in 100% juice if canned), drained well

1. Preheat oven to 310°F and grease muffin pan with coconut oil or insert paper muffin cups.

2. Using an electric mixer, blend together butter, honey, yogurt and eggs until smooth.

3. In a separate bowl, mix coconut, almond flour, baking powder and salt with a wire whisk until all chunks are blended together well.

4. Combine all ingredients accept for the pineapple in a large bowl and mix together well with the whisk.

5. Spoon pineapple into each muffin cup until the bottom is filled. Using an ice cream scoop, drop one scoop of the muffin batter into each cup, covering up the pineapple.

6. Bake for 30 minutes or until tops of muffins are golden brown. Cool completely and serve plain or cut muffins in half and spread with yogurt cheese or butter.

Mini-Berry Pies

I found these great rainbow-colored silicone muffin cups while searching for Christmas presents for my son who loves to help me in the kitchen. I used them to bake these mini-pies, but you can also use conventional muffin tins with paper cups. You may have to adjust the baking time depending on what you use, but they are sure to satisfy the sweet tooth either way!

Yield: 12 muffin-sized pies

Crust
6 tablespoons butter, melted
2 tablespoons agave
1 cup blanched almond flour

Filling
1 pint heavy whipping cream
3 tablespoons agave
6 ounces fresh organic blueberries
6 ounces fresh organic raspberries

1. Preheat oven to 250°F. Line muffin pans with paper cups, or if using silicone, grease lightly with coconut oil.

2. In a medium-sized mixing bowl, combine butter, agave and almond flour until well blended. Scoop about one tablespoon into each muffin cup and spread evenly along inside and bottom, using your fingers for best results.

3. Bake crusts for about 10 minutes or until crispy and golden brown.

4. Meanwhile, in a large mixing bowl, combine whipping cream and agave and blend on high with electric beaters until soft peaks form. (Continued on next page)

5. After cooling crust slightly, spoon whipped cream into muffin cups and top with berries as desired. Eat right out of the cups with a spoon, or turn over into bowls.

4th of July Pie Variation! Double ingredients, bake in a rectangular dish, and layer berries on top of whipped cream to represent the American flag.

Coconut Macaroons

Macaroons make a great snack and are easy to bag up as a take-along treat. All of my kids love these in either cupcake size or bite-sized portions. Used with permission from Lucy's SCD Cookbook, p. 86.

Yield: 15 cup cake sized macaroons

6 egg whites
1/4 teaspoon sea salt
1/2 cup honey
2 teaspoons pure sugar-free vanilla extract
2 1/2 cups unsweetened, finely shredded coconut

1. Preheat oven to 300°F. Grease muffin tins or silicone cups with coconut oil.

2. Beat the egg whites and salt with electric mixer on medium speed until stiff.

3. Gently fold in the honey, vanilla, and coconut using a large rubber or silicone spatula.

4. Using an ice-cream scoop, fill each paper cup about 3/4 of the way full.

5. Bake for 25-30 minutes, or until tops of macaroons are golden brown.

Apple-Cinnamon Almond Cookies

These soft, chewy and only slightly sweet cookies make a great after school snack in addition to being a healthy dessert.

Yield: About 15 cookies

4 tablespoons butter, melted
1/2 teaspoon pure vanilla extract
1/2 cup agave or honey
1 teaspoon cinnamon
1/8 teaspoon sea salt
1/2 teaspoon Ener-G baking powder (or 1/4 teaspoon baking soda)
1/2 cup raisins (optional, *S*)
1/2 apple, peeled and grated, or 1/2 cup no-sugar added applesauce *S*
2 cups blanched almond flour

1. Preheat oven to 300°F. Mix butter, vanilla, agave, cinnamon, salt, and baking powder with a wire whisk in a medium-sized bowl.

2. Add raisins and apple and mix together well. Mix in almond flour with a wooden spoon until flour has absorbed all the liquid and can be formed into ball.

3. Using a small scoop or tablespoon, place balls of mix onto an ungreased cookie sheet. Flatten cookies with the back of a spoon or fork.

4. Bake for 35 minutes or until cookies are a dark golden brown. Cool completely on a cooling rack before serving.

Swedish Cardamom* Mini Loaves

These mini loaves make great holiday gifts or contribution to the holiday dessert table. Some of my favorite holiday memories come from baking cardamom bread with my mom and sisters. Since our traditional wheat flour recipe is now taboo for my kids, I came up with this grain-free version which goes great with a cup of decaf chai!

Yield: 4 mini-loaves

1 cup honey
½ cup grapeseed oil
4 large eggs
1 tablespoon pure vanilla extract
4 tablespoons melted, unsalted butter
5 cups blanched, finely ground almond flour (www.nutsonline.com)
4 teaspoons Ener-G baking powder OR 2 teaspoons baking soda
1 teaspoon sea salt
4 teaspoons ground cardamom
1 cup raisins, chopped into small bits (optional, may require Sucraid)

1. Preheat oven to 350°F. Grease loaf pans with grapeseed oil or butter.

2. In a medium bowl, combine honey, grapeseed oil, eggs, vanilla and melted butter with a wire whisk and blend well.

3. In a large bowl, combine almond flour, baking powder, sea salt and cardamom until thoroughly blended. Add wet mixture from medium bowl and mix well.

4. Pour batter evenly into greased loaf pans and bake for 30 minutes or until tops begins to brown.

5. Carefully remove pan and cover bread with foil. Return to oven and bake an additional 20 minutes or until inserted toothpick comes out clean.

6. Cool bread about five minutes and remove from pan to cool completely on wire cooking racks. The cooler the bread is, the easier it will be to slice without crumbling.

7. Serve with softened butter or cream cheese.

Apple Pie

My daughter adored me for making her this special separate apple pie for Thanksgiving. The almond flour crust is easier than handmade traditional crust in my opinion. Whipped cream topping is optional.

Yield: 4 Servings

For Crust
1/4 cup blanched almond flour
1/4 cup melted unsalted butter
1/8 teaspoon sea salt

Filling
2 cups apples, peeled, cored and sliced (Granny Smith work best) *S*
1/4 cup blanched almond flour
1/4 teaspoon nutmeg
1/4 teaspoon cinnamon
1/4 teaspoon
1/2 cup agave

1. Preheat oven to 325°F.

2. Mix together almond flour and butter and press evenly into bottom and sides of a 9-inch pie dish (or 2 4-inch ramekins as shown in picture).

3. Bake the crust for about 10 minutes or until light brown. Place on cooling rack, leaving oven on.

4. Mix filling ingredients in a large bowl. Pour mixture into pie dish or ramekins.

5. Bake for 40-50 minutes or until brown and bubbly. Serve warm or cool with homemade whipping cream sweetened with agave.

Appendix

Roanne King

One-Week Sample Menu

The recipes for these meals can be found in section 3-Recipes according to meal type. Most of these recipes are designed for use **after** *successfully completing all phases of the* Induction Diet (see chapter 5) *to determine individual tolerance levels for starches, sugars and milk products.*

SUNDAY
 Breakfast
 • *French Toast* and Fresh Fruit*
 Lunch
 • Tuna Melt*
  Sweet 'N Crunchy Salad
 Dinner
 • Chicken and Lima Bean Soup
 • Green Salad with Tomato and Shredded Carrots

MONDAY
 Breakfast
 • Breakfast Crepes
 Lunch
 • Chicken and Lima Bean Soup w/ Grilled Cheese*
 Dinner
 • Turkey Meatloaf with Mashed Cauliflower
 • Spinach and Strawberry Salad

TUESDAY
 Breakfast
 • Fried Eggs and Almond Bread Toast*
 Lunch
 • Cucumber, Cheese and Turkey Sandwiches
 • Fresh blueberries
 Dinner
 • Salmon Fillets with Dill and Lemon
 • Steamed green beans and salad

WEDNESDAY
 Breakfast

- Rainbow Scrambled Eggs
- Turkey sausage and sliced strawberries

Lunch
- Turkey, Cream Cheese and Spinach Wrap

Dinner
- Fried Chicken Patties and Steamed Broccoli

THURSDAY
Breakfast
- Rise and Shine Smoothie

Lunch
- Cottage Cheese with Fruit or Tomato Slices

Dinner
- Creamy Chicken Casserole

FRIDAY
Breakfast
- Almond and Coconut Pancakes

Lunch
- Celery Slices with Tuna and/or Almond Butter

Dinner
- Ground Turkey with Zucchini and Carrots

SATURDAY
Breakfast
- Almond Cereal with Fruit

Lunch
- Spinach, Carrot and Strawberry Salad
- Apple Slices and Almond Butter

Dinner
- Zucchini Lasagna
- Steamed Carrots

*use almond or coconut bread

One-Week Shopping List

Dairy

- Plain yogurt (no added starch or maltodextrin)
- 2 dozen eggs
- Milk
- Mozzarella and cheddar cheese in blocks
- Cream cheese
- Cottage Cheese
- Heavy whipping cream
- Butter
- Daisy sour cream

Fish, Pork and Poultry

- Large bag frozen chicken tenders
- 4-6 Salmon fillets
- 4 pounds ground turkey
- Turkey breast

Canned/Dry Goods

- Dry white butter beans
- 64-ounce bottle 100%Tomato juice
- Albacore Tuna (in water or oil only)
- Coconut Milk (no sugar or starch fillers)

Fruits and Vegetables

- Red, yellow and orange bell peppers
- White mushrooms
- Alfalfa sprouts
- Broccoli crowns
- Whole cauliflower
- Apples
- Bananas
- Strawberries
- Red, seedless grapes
- Celery

- Oranges
- Cucumber
- Avocado
- Tomatoes
- Baby spinach leaves
- Baby carrots
- Kale
- Yellow onion
- Garlic
- Leafy green lettuce
- Lemons
- Zucchini
- Frozen blueberries

Pantry Items

- Dried oregano, basil, thyme, rosemary
- Whole, raw almonds
- Red wine vinegar
- Parmesan cheese
- Almond flour
- Unsweetened, shredded coconut
- Flax oil
- Dried dill weed
- Sea salt
- Black pepper
- Olive oil
- Coconut oil
- Grapeseed oil
- Slivered almonds
- Pure vanilla extract
- Pure fruit jam
- Ener-G Baking Powder
- Raisins
- Honey
- Agave Nectar (organic when possible)

Resource List

For updates and more recipes, please follow my blog at www.csidrecipes.com

LUCY'S KITCHEN SHOP
LucysKitchenShop.com
Call toll free 888-484-2126
Outside U.S. 360-647-2279
Email lucy@lucyskitchenshop.com
Products: *Almond flour, shredded coconut, yogurt maker, yogurt starter*

NUTS.COM
Nuts.com
800-558-6887
Products: *Almond flour, coconut, agave syrup, whole almonds, coconut flour*

ENERGETIC NUTRITION
EnergeticNutrition.com
Online supplements shipped around the globe including systemic enzymes, digestive enzymes, multivitamin and mineral supplements from various, trusted brands.

NATURE'S SUNSHINE
NaturesSunshine.com
800-223-8225
Products: *liquid chlorophyll, food enzymes, marshmallow root capsules, probiotics, Sunshine Heroes Probiotic Power, Sunshine Heroes Papaya Enzymes, magnesium complex*

SHAKLEE
Shaklee.com
800-742-5533
Products: *Incredivites™ Chewable Multivitamins, Shakleebaby™ Multivitamin & Multimineral Powder, household cleaners, prebiotics and probiotics*

KIRKMAN
KirkmanLabs.com
800-245-8282
Products: *Carb Digest™ with Isogest®, EnZym-Complete/DPP-IV™ II with Isogest®*

GLORY BEE FOODS
GloryBee.com
Products: *shredded coconut, agave syrup*

Sucraid Information
Sucraid.net

CSID Links
CSIDcares.org
CSIDinfo.com
CSIDRecipes.com (not affiliated with CSIDinfo or CSIDCares)

PALEO BOOKS
I've found the Paleo Diet reflects the CSID diet more closely than any other. These books have been most helpful in educating me on the reasons for Paleo. The recipes are top-notch and better than anything I could create on my own.

Against All Grain books by Danielle Walker
Practical Paleo books by Diane Sanfilippo, BS, NC
21-Day Sugar Detox by Diane Sanfilippo, BS, NC

Bibliography

Ayers, Art. Breastfeeding Decreases Celiac and Diabetes: Weaning After First Foods Protects Against Autoimmune Diseases. December 26, 2008. http://pregnancychildbirth.suite101.com/article.cfm/breastfeeding_decreases_celiac_and_diabetes (accessed March 27, 2009).

Bager, Jodi, and Lass, Jenny. "Grain Free Gourmet." North Vancouver: Whitecap Books, 2005.

Bager, Jodi and Lass, Jenny. "Everyday Grain-Free Gourmet". North Vancouver: Whitecap Books, 2008.

Balch, Phyllis A. "Prescription for Nutritional Healing." New York: Penguin Putnam Inc., 2002.

Bowden, Jonny Ph.D., C.N.S. "The 150 Healthiest Foods on Earth." Beverly: Fair Winds Press, 2007.

Brostoff, Jonathan, MD, and Gamilin Linda. "Food Allergies and Food Intolerance." Rochester: Healing Arts Press, 2000.

Brown, Susan E. MD, and Larry Jr. Trivirieri. "The Acid Alkaline Food Guide." Garden City Park: Square One Publishers, 2006.

CSID Parent Support Group. www.csidinfo.com (accessed March 25, 2009).

Czapp, Katherine. Against the Grain. 2006. http://www.westonaprice.org/moderndiseases/gluten-intolerance.html (accessed March 26, 2009).

Duyff, Roberta Larson. "American Dietetic Association Complete Food and Nutrition Guide". Revised and updated 3rd Edition. The American Dietetic Association, 2006.

Fife, Bruce C.N., N.D. "The Coconut Oil Miracle." New York: Penguin Group, 2004.

Fife, Bruce. "Cooking With Coconut Flour." Colorado Springs: Piccadily Books, Ltd., 2005.

Gott, Peter, H, M.D. "Dr. Gott's No Flour, No Sugar Diet." Warner Books., 2006.

Gottschall, Elaine, B.A., M. Sc. "Breaking the Vicious Cycle." Baltimore, Ontario: Kirkton Press Ltd., 2004.

Holt, Stephen M.D. "Natural Ways to Digestive Health." New York: M. Evans and Company, Inc., 2000.

Joneja, Janice Vickerstaff, PhD, RD. "Dealing With Food Allergies in Babies and Children." Boulder: Bull Publishing Company, 2007.

Kliment, Felicia Drury. "The Acid Alkaline Balance Diet". Revised Edition. McGraw-Hill Books, 2010.

Mayo Clinic. "Mayo Clinic on Digestive Health." New York: Kensington Publishing Corporation, 2000.

MedicineNet. 1996-2009. www.medicinenet.com/celiac_disease/article.htm (accessed March 19, 2009).

Miller, Janette Brand. McVeagh, Patricia. "Human Milk Ogliosaccharides: 130 Reasons to Breastfeed." *British Journal of Nutrition,* 1999. Pp 333-335.

National Digestive Diseases Information Clearinghouse. Celiac Disease. http://digestive.niddk.nih.gov/ddiseases/pubs/celiac/ (accessed March 12, 2009).

Peikin, Steven R. M.D. "Gastrointestinal Health." New York: HarperCollins Publishers Inc., 1999.

Prasad, Ramad. "Recipes for the Specific Carbohydrate Diet." Beverly: Fairwinds Press, 2008.

Ramacher, Sandra. "Healing Foods: Cooking for Celiacs, Colitis, Crohn's and IBS. Elephant Publishing, 2007.

Rehmeyer, Julie J. "Milk Therapy: Breast Milk Compounds Could Be a Tonic for Adult Ills." *Science News.* 170.24. December 9, 2006. p. 376.Retrieved from Infotrac Custome 750 Journals on February 1, 2012.

Rosenfeld, Isadore M.D. "Doctor, What Should I Eat?" New York: Random House, Inc., 1995.

Rosset, Lucy. "Lucy's Specific Carbohydrate Diet Cookbook." Bellingham: Lucy's Kitchen Shop, 2000.

Tweed, Vera. "Digestive Defenders: pint-sized probiotics play a giant role in immune health." Better Nutrition. August 2011. Retrieved from InfoTrac Custom 750 Journals, February 1, 2012.

Vasey, Christopher N.D. "The Acid-Alkaline Diet for Optimum Health." Rochester: Healing Arts Press, 2003.

Walker, Marsha, RN, IBCLC. "Supplementation of the Breastfed Baby: Just One Bottle Won't Hurt, or Will It?" N.D.

Yaron, Ruth. "Super Baby Food." Peckville: F.J. Roberts Publishing Company, 2003.

Young, Robert O. PhD, and Young Shelley Redford. "The pH Miracle: Balance Your Diet, Reclaim Your Health." New York: Warner Books, 2002.

Notes:

Notes:

Notes:

Notes:

Notes:

Notes:

Index

Roanne King

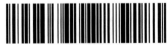

44476275R00111

Made in the USA
Lexington, KY
10 July 2019